Body Therapy
& Facial Work

Body Therapy & Facial Work

Electrical Treatments for Beauty Therapists

3rd edition

Mo Rosser

Hodder Arnold

A MEMBER OF THE HODDER HEADLINE GROUP

To my delightful grandchildren Zachary, Joshua, Hannah and Isobel

Orders: please contact Bookpoint Ltd, 130 Milton Park, Abingdon, Oxon OX14 4SB.
Telephone: (44) 01235 827720. Fax: (44) 01235 400454. Lines are open from 9.00–5.00,
Monday to Saturday, with a 24 hour message answering service. You can also order through
our website www.hoddereducation.co.uk

If you have any comments to make about this, or any of our other titles, please send them to
educationenquiries@hodder.co.uk

British Library Cataloguing in Publication Data
A catalogue record for this title is available from the British Library

ISBN-10: 0 340 926 058
ISBN-13: 978 0 340 926 055

First Edition Published 1996
Second Edition Published 2004
This Edition Published 2006
Impression number   10 9 8 7 6 5 4 3 2
Year   2010 2009 2008 2007 2006

Copyright © 1996, 2004, 2006 Mo Rosser

Hodder Headline's policy is to use papers that are natural, renewable and
recyclable products and made from wood grown in sustainable forests.
The logging and manufacturing processes are expected to conform to the
environmental regulations of the country of origin.

Cover photo from Colin Anderson/Brand X Pictures/Getty Images

Artwork by: Mike Parsons, Barking Dog Art
Typeset by Charon Tec Ltd, Chennai, India
www.charontec.com
Printed in Great Britain from Hodder Arnold, an imprint of Hodder Education, a member of the
Hodder Headline Group, 338 Euston Road, London NW1 3BH by CPI Bath

Contents

Acknowledgments

I am indebted to the following for their help and advice during the preparation of this book: Greta Couldridge, for meticulously reading and advising on all aspects of the text, Peter Thompson for his computer skills and Suzanne and Gwyn Rosser for all their help and support.

To the following for specialist advice: Dr Rosemary J. S. Jones, Senior Research Fellow, Bristol University (Chapter 6), Mr J. Hawk, Consultant Dermatologist, St Thomas's Hospital, London (Chapter 7) and Vanessa Puttnick, Technical Director, The Hairdressing and Beauty Equipment Centre, London N7 for technical advice. Thanks also to Jorge Centofanti, Marketing Director, Ultratone, London W1H for reading and giving advice on Chapter 9.

Thank you to the following companies for supplying and allowing us to reproduce photographs: The Hairdressing and Beauty Equipment Centre, 262 Holloway Road, London N7; Ultratone, 36 George Street, London W1H; Guinot, The Clock House, Ascot, Berkshire; Thalgo, Thalgo House, Blackheath Village, London SE3; Sorisa, Bellissima House, 212 Northenden Road, Sale, Manchester, M33 2PA; Tansun, Spectrum House, Unit 1, Ridgeacre Road, West Bromwich, West Midlands B71 1BW and Carlton Group, Carlton House, Commerce Way, Lancing, West Sussex BN1S 8TA.

The author and publishers would like to thank the following for the use of photographs in this volume: p14 Edward Webb/Rex Features, pp21, 34, 36, 76, 103, 104, 109, 115–118, 126, 136, 143, 152, 161, 228, 259, 274 The Carlton Group, p29 David Scharf/Science Photo Library, p50 Belle Sante, p90 Photodisc, pp105, 130, 134, 138 (top left and right), 168, 217 Sorisa, p138 (bottom) CACI International, pp176, 192, 209 Ultratone, pp223, 238 Tansun, p257 Profimedia. CZ s.r.o/Alamy, p271 Andre Jenny/Alamy.

Introduction

This book has been revised to meet the new standards and requirements of the various awarding bodies relating to electrical treatments for the face and body. It will provide the student with the necessary underpinning knowledge to select appropriate treatments and the skills instruction to operate the equipment safely. The information will explain the science relating to each treatment, the application technique and the effects. This detail will enable the therapist to discuss and fully explain the selected treatment with each client and to carry out the procedure in a safe and effective manner.

Emphasis is placed on the responsibilities and legal requirements of every therapist under the Health, Safety and Hygiene Acts. These are very important issues which must be adhered to in order to protect therapists, clients and other salon personnel from injury and cross infection.

In addition to having detailed knowledge and understanding of all the available treatments, the competent therapist must have the professionalism, confidence and personality to deal with the broader aspects of her role. Guidance is provided for developing good communication skills and for dealing with a wide range of clients with differing personalities. Contraindications and contra-actions are explained and advice given on client consultation, assessment, planning outcomes and selecting effective appropriate treatments. Consideration is given to the timing and costing of treatments, together with post-treatment observation, feedback and home advice.

The book is broadly divided into four sections.

Health, safety and hygiene issues

This section covers the legal requirements relating to health and safety in the workplace. It identifies potential hazards and risks and suggests ways of eliminating them. Information is provided on the role of the inspectorate, responsibilities of employers, managers, supervisors and employees under these acts. This section offers guidance for legal and safe practice.

Ethics, consultation and care of the client

This deals with developing the highest standards of personal behaviour and projecting an efficient, professional and caring image. It includes consultation and assessment; preparation of the client, therapist and the working area; dealing with and adapting to a wide range of clients; the recording of data and the importance of confidentiality; an explanation of contraindications, contra-actions, feedback and aftercare.

Underpinning science

This covers basic scientific principles, describes the different currents used in the treatments and explains the mode by which treatments are effective.

The application of individual treatments

This section includes the underpinning knowledge and skills instruction for each treatment. The information covers relevant scientific theory, the uses, effects, contraindications, dangers, safety precautions, treatment technique, contra-actions, feedback and aftercare.

The aim of the book is to provide the student with comprehensive information which will facilitate her understanding of electrotherapy and enable her to practise effectively and safely. Revision notes are included in the text and questions are added at the end of each chapter.

Assessment guidance is provided covering the evidence required to succeed and demonstrate competence. Knowledge and skill requirements, performance criteria and the range statements are included.

The information will enable the student to self study and acquire an understanding of each electrical treatment. The step by step practical instructions provide the guidance necessary to carry out the treatments efficiently and safely to commercially acceptable standards and timescales.

Electrical treatments are effective with visually obvious results, they are therefore among the most popular treatments offered in beauty salons, health spas/ clinics, leisure centres, sports complexes, etc. The competent therapist with a caring attitude, who maintains high ethical standards and projects a positive, professional image, will always be in demand. She will establish an excellent reputation among colleagues and clients and will contribute to the efficiency and success of the salon. A qualification in electrotherapy offers many opportunities for an exciting and rewarding career.

Learning and Assessment Guidance

As you pursue this course of study and practice, the information provided in this book will enable you to:

1 Communicate effectively, pleasantly and professionally with colleagues and clients.

2 Acquire the knowledge and understanding of how and why electrical treatments work.

3 Assess the client's needs; select, advise and discuss the most suitable treatments.

4 Gain the skills necessary to perform electrical treatments safely and effectively on different types of client for a variety of conditions of the face and body.

Learning

Knowledge and understanding

You will require background knowledge to be competent in your work and to be able to explain the effects and benefits of the treatment to your clients.

Health and safety legislation

You must understand the health, safety and welfare requirements related to your work. These will enable you to practise safely and protect yourself, colleagues and clients from harm. The relevant health, safety and welfare issues are discussed in the next chapter together with local authority regulations. These are legal requirements and are concerned with identifying and rectifying the hazards and risks in your place of work.

Remember that as a therapist you carry the responsibility of ensuring your own safety and the safety and welfare of the clients and others who come to the salon. In these days of litigation you may well be sued if anyone sustains an injury or is harmed due to your negligence. Therefore it is vital that all safety requirements are adhered to and accurate records kept of all risk assessments or incidents that occur.

Without doubt, treatments using electrical equipment pose the greatest risks of any treatments in the salon. It is therefore crucial that you fully understand and learn all the safety issues related to the equipment, the practices and the precautions necessary to avoid any problems. You must also learn important emergency procedures such as fire drill and first aid.

It is very important that you maintain the highest standards of hygiene and cleanliness. If you consistently maintain high standards, this will become normal practice. However if you allow your standards to slip you will find it difficult to raise them for the assessment and you will be a danger to the clients and a liability in the salon. Throughout the working day, the highest standards of hygiene must be practised to prevent the spread of diseases and to protect staff, clients and others from cross infection and infestation.

Hygiene relates to your own personal appearance and hygiene practices such as a clean laundered overall daily, neat appearance, short well-manicured nails, minimum of jewellery, frequent bathing, hand washing before touching the client and after each treatment, etc. It includes salon hygiene such as a clean well-ventilated, adequately-lit salon; clean boil-washed linen, robes and towels for each client; clean bedroll and clean disinfected equipment; prompt and safe disposal of waste into covered waste bins, etc. It also covers client hygiene such as taking a shower before treatment; cleansing the areas of the body that are to be treated; checking for and dealing with any contraindications, etc.

Communication

You must be able to communicate effectively and pleasantly with all types of people. You may need to adapt your style to suit the client; it is your duty to make the client feel at ease and relaxed.

You must recognise the importance of listening to the client and discussing her needs and aspirations.

You must be able to explain the benefits and advantages of the treatment that you are proposing.

Anatomy and physiology

A knowledge of the structure and function of the body is necessary, as this will enable you to identify the structures you are working over and understand the effects produced on the body systems.

It will help you to learn this subject if you try to visualise the tissues underneath your hands as you examine and cleanse the area:

- Your hands are in contact with the skin; what is the skin composed of?

- Could you draw and label a section through the skin?

- How would you identify the different skin types and conditions?

- Under the skin is the subcutaneous layer, what is it made of?

- Under the subcutaneous layer lie the muscles, can you name these muscles and give their action?

- Under the muscles lie the bones connected at joints, can you name the bones and the joints?

During assessment you may be required to give the name, the position and the action of certain superficial muscles. These are covered in this book together with the name and location of the lymph nodes.

Unfortunately this book does not include detailed anatomy, but some topics are revised to help you understand the treatments. Detailed anatomy is covered in *Body Massage* by Mo Rosser.

Equipment

You must ensure that you are familiar with all equipment that you use:

- Always read the manufacturers' instructions. Ensure that you understand all the detail. If you do not, contact the company and ask for an explanation.

- Pay particular attention to all the safety features.

- Check the machine before each use; it must be clean and in sound condition.

- Check that the cable and leads have no breaks in the insulation; there should be no exposed wires.

- Ensure that the cable is not trailing over the floor or working area.

- Check that the cable is firmly held at the plug end and in the machine; check that the terminals are safely and securely engaged in their correct sockets.

- Identify the type of current produced.

- Ensure that you are familiar with all the controls and connections.

- Ensure that you fully understand what is happening when you make any adjustment to any of the controls.

- Test the current on yourself before applying it to the client.

- Ensure that all the intensity controls are at zero before switching on.

- Clean the equipment according to health and safety requirements after use.

Guide to study

Some of you will find study and learning easy and pleasurable; it is always exciting to learn new things, particularly if the course is one you have chosen and success means that there will be an interesting and rewarding career ahead. Others may find study difficult, especially if there has been a long gap in the learning process or there is little prior knowledge of the subject matter. The material in this book has been carefully organized so that you can learn one step at a time. I hope that you find it interesting and easy to follow.

Many of you will have established your own way of study but those of you who find it difficult may find the following pointers helpful:

■ Prepare for study, preferably in a quiet place; have some paper and a pen beside you.

■ Select a small piece of text. Read it through from beginning to the end; this will give you an idea of what it's all about.

■ Take one or two paragraphs at a time and read them through several times until you really understand the detail.

■ Write down the important points and the definitions which you must know.

■ Now close the book and try and remember the detail. Test yourself mentally then write down the main facts.

■ Move on to the next section and repeat the above process. Do this until you reach the end of your selected text.

■ Turn to the summary at the end of the chapter. Did you remember all that is written here?

Now try and answer the relevant questions. Write down your answers as this will help you to remember and recall the information.

The first set of questions at the end of each chapter have been designed as written questions. You will find the answers in the text. If you do not know the answer you will need to search for it and read it again and again. This will consolidate the facts and help you to remember them.

The second set of questions are designed as oral questions and the answers are provided at the end of the book. You may wish to study these with a partner so that you can test each other.

> When you are studying the text, select small chunks, read these several times, write your own notes on key points, use the summaries, ask yourself questions and answer them.

Assessment

Any assessment is an opportunity for you to show how able you are. You will provide evidence of this ability to the assessor, who will judge your performance against the standards set by the awarding body.

Throughout the course you will be required to provide various types of evidence which the assessor will judge and decide whether you are competent and capable of working to the National Standards.

Do not be apprehensive when you come to be assessed. Providing you have worked consistently, you will have gained the skills and knowledge required to succeed. You may decide when you are ready to be assessed. Each assessment is your chance to demonstrate how good you are, and to provide evidence of your knowledge and skill.

This book has been designed to help you achieve your goals. Ask your tutor or teaching centre for a copy of the unit you are studying. Do this at the beginning of the course. Read each section carefully. The unit will tell you exactly what you need to know. Do not be put off or be apprehensive as you read it; remember that you are going to acquire this knowledge one step at a time. Each awarding body will specify their own requirements but they must all work towards the same National Standards.

The Hairdressing and Beauty Industry Authority (HABIA) identifies the skill needs in these industries and sets the standards of competence, knowledge and understanding required to meet these needs. Units can be downloaded from the web site of the awarding body; your college or tutor will have this information.

The HABIA website is www.habia.org.

Remember you are responsible for providing evidence of your competence; your tutor or assessor will help you by providing guidance and support. Make sure that you understand what is required of you.

'If you know where you are going, you are more able to help yourself get there.'

Discuss the unit with your assessor, develop and agree assessment plans. Make sure that you understand the procedure and what evidence is to be presented at each assessment.

You may have past experience and achievements which may count towards the competence for this unit. This is usually referred to as accreditation of prior learning. Remember to ask if past employment or training can be taken into account.

Before undertaking any assessment, the assessor must provide you with a list of criteria and the range statements. These will inform you of the knowledge and skill competences required to succeed.

The assessor should read through the criteria and range statements with you and offer support and advice. Make sure you understand everything that is said and ask for clarification if in doubt.

Practical assessment

Your assessor will watch you working and will assess your performance against national standards. You and the assessor will decide on the type of assessment and where the assessment is to take place. Evidence may be collected when you are treating a client in college or in the workplace. You will be assessed several times throughout the course on different equipment and different types of client.

At every assessment you must ensure that you cover the following:

- Prepare yourself to meet hygiene standards.

- Prepare the area and ensure the correct environmental conditions in accordance with HSE recommendations.

- Carry out a consultation; assess the client's needs and expectations; carry out a skin and facial contour analysis for facial work, or a posture, muscle tone, fat/cellulite analysis for body work.

- Select the most beneficial treatment; discuss and agree the treatment with the client. Prepare the client for treatment; check for contraindications; carry out a skin sensitivity test (sharp/blunt and hot/cold); cleanse the area.

- Carry out the treatment within the safety standards and correct procedures.

- Check for contra-actions and take appropriate action.

- Obtain feedback and advise aftercare.

- Help the client off the bed and into the changing room.

- Cleanse/disinfect/sterilize the equipment as appropriate.

You may be questioned by the assessor during or after the performance. The assessor should indicate whether you may stop the treatment when answering questions. Continue working if you are not told to stop.

As previously explained additional questions and answers have been included in this edition. They are compiled as oral questions which you may be asked during a practical assessment.

Written assessment

Your knowledge and understanding may be assessed through written questions, special assignments, projects or case studies.

Some suggestions for topics suitable for projects are:

a. Are the health, safety and hygiene requirements being upheld in your college or workplace? Discuss the potential hazards and risks and the action that must be taken to avoid them.

   Information can be obtained from the Health and Safety Executive (HSE). Web site: www.hse.gov.uk.

b. Discuss the safety requirements and legalities which you must consider when using six named types of equipment and explain why some pose greater dangers than others.

c. Compare and contrast the effects, ease of use and client satisfaction when using three microcurrent machines from different manufacturers. This could be supported by manufacturers' claims, video evidence, photographs, record cards, etc.

After every assessment you will be given feedback by your assessor who will discuss your performance with you and tell you if you have been successful or unsuccessful.

If you have been successful this will be recorded. If you have not been successful you will be offered further training. You have the right to appeal against an assessor's decision; your training centre will inform you of the procedure to follow should you wish to do so. You will find it helpful to keep your own written record of each piece of evidence as you provide it and an account of every practical assessment. Include the comments and advice of the assessor.

All the evidence you produce to demonstrate competence, knowledge and understanding is recorded and collected into a portfolio of evidence which is finally presented for certification.

Remember, to succeed you must:

- Satisfy all evidence requirements.
- Meet all performance criteria.
- Include all aspects of the range.
- Meet all knowledge and understanding requirements.

Underpinning Knowledge

1 Health, Safety and Welfare

Health, Safety and Welfare at Work

Health and safety is about preventing any person sustaining injury, being harmed in any way or becoming ill at work. It involves following correct, safe procedures and taking every possible precaution to protect everyone in the workplace.

OBJECTIVES

After you have studied this chapter you will be able to:

1 Understand the legal requirements under the Health and Safety at Work Act.

2 Distinguish between hazard and risk.

3 Explain the role of the Health and Safety Executive (HSE).

4 List the actions that may be taken by the HSE.

5 Differentiate between health, safety and welfare issues in the workplace.

6 Discuss the ways of protecting everyone in the workplace from exposure to hazardous substances.

7 Explain the safety considerations related to electrical equipment.

8 Understand the importance of reporting injuries, diseases and dangerous occurrences.

9 Describe the importance of administering first aid in the work place.

10 Describe the correct techniques for lifting.

11 State the precautions which must be in place to meet fire regulations.

12 Carry out a risk assessment.

Hazards and risks

Health and safety laws and regulations apply to you and everyone working with you. These will include employers, managers, supervisors, employees, self-employed, full or part-time, paid or unpaid workers.

Health and safety issues refer to hazards and risks in the workplace and how to eliminate them.

Definitions

Hazard means anything that has the potential to cause harm.

Risk is the chance, great or small, that someone will be harmed by the hazard.

Do not ignore any hazard or risk in your workplace. Rectify the problem or report it to a senior person who can.

Health and Safety at Work Act 1974

This is the main legislation covering health and safety in the workplace, other safety regulations and codes of practice come under this main act.

This act states that:

Employers/managers have a legal duty to ensure, so far as is reasonably practicable, the health, safety and welfare of all persons at work, that is all employees and other persons on the premises, such as contractors and clients.

The Health and Safety Executive provides information and publications on all aspects of health and safety regulations, implementing directives from the European Commission which used to be known as the six pack. These cover a wide range of health, safety and welfare issues. Those relevant to the therapist are dealt with in this text.

The Health and Safety Executive (HSE)

This is a body of people appointed to enforce health and safety law. Inspectors from the Health and Safety Executive or from your Local Authority have the statutory right to inspect your workplace at any time, with or without prior notice. During the visit the inspector will be looking at the premises, the working environment and the work practices. The inspector will check that you are complying with health and safety law and will assess whether there are any hazards or risks to the health, safety or welfare of anyone on the premises.

The inspectors can:

- inspect all aspects relating to health, safety and welfare
- take photographs
- ask questions or talk to anyone in the salon
- investigate any complaint
- offer guidance and advice.

The inspector will ensure that those in charge have arrangements in place for consulting with, training and informing all staff on all matters relating to health, safety and welfare. All staff will be given the opportunity to speak to the inspector privately should they wish to do so. The inspector will provide information and highlight areas of concern to the employers and will also explain why enforcement action is to be taken.

If a breach of the law is found, the inspector will decide what action to take. The action will depend on the severity of the problem.

Actions which may be taken by HSE inspectors

1 **Informal notice:** If the problem is a minor one, the inspector may simply explain what must be done to comply with the law. If asked he will confirm any advice in writing.

2 **Improvement notice:** If the problem is more serious, the inspector may issue an improvement notice. This will state what needs to be done and the time limit by which it must be done. At least 21 days must be allowed for corrective action to be taken.

3 **Prohibition notice:** If the problem poses a serious risk, the inspector may give notice to stop the activity immediately and not allow it to be resumed until corrective action is taken. The notice will explain why such action is necessary.

4 **Prosecution:** A failure to act upon an improvement or prohibition notice may result in prosecution. The courts have the power to impose unlimited fines and in some severe cases, imprisonment.

An employer has the right of appeal to an industrial tribunal when an improvement or prohibition notice is served should the employer disagree with it or feel that it is unjust. The instructions on how to appeal appear on the back of the notice.

The Therapist's Role in Health and Safety

The employer/manager/supervisor is responsible for the management and control of health, safety and welfare issues which will ensure a safe environment for all persons working in or attending the salon/clinic. However all therapists at work also have a duty under the Health and Safety Act.

Employer/manager/supervisor responsibilities

The Act of 1974 and the new regulations mean that employers must, by law, provide a safe working environment for all members of the workforce including those with disabilities and other persons using their premises.

Employers/managers/supervisors are required to:

- Provide a safe working environment; they must recognize hazards or risks, and take the appropriate actions to minimize or eliminate them.

- Have a written health and safety policy which sets out how these issues are managed.

- Assess the risks which may arise from work activities.

- Record the findings of the risk assessment.

- Consult with colleagues and employees regarding health and safety issues.

■ Provide health and safety information, training and supervision for all employees.

Employee responsibilities

Employees are required to:
■ Take reasonable care to avoid harm to themselves or to others by their behaviour or working practices.

■ Cooperate and help employers/managers to meet the statutory requirements.

■ Refrain from misusing or interfering with anything provided to protect the health, safety and welfare of all persons as required by the Health and Safety at Work Act.

To comply with these requirements you must:
■ Not put yourself or others at risk by your actions.

■ Abide by salon rules and regulations.

■ Know who is responsible for what in the salon and to whom you should report problems.

■ Always adopt good working practices and follow correct procedures.

■ Be alert to and do not ignore any hazard which may pose a risk to yourself or to others and promptly take the appropriate action to minimize or eliminate the risk. If you are unable to, or unsure of how to quickly deal with a hazard, then you must *report the situation* to someone else immediately.

Seek advice from a supervisor or someone qualified to deal with the situation.

■ Be competent in selecting appropriate treatments and in administering them correctly and safely to the clients.

■ Follow the correct technique for all treatments, understand the effects, and be alert to contraindications and contra-actions.

■ Adopt high professional standards of dress and appearance.

Ensure that your actions do not put others at risk:
■ Maintain the highest standards of personal and salon hygiene.

■ Report faulty equipment to the person responsible for dealing with these issues.

■ Do not ignore any hazard or risk, make sure that corrective action is taken.

■ Keep a record of and report any problems that you have identified and rectified.

■ Inform your supervisor and colleagues and be prepared to discuss issues of health and safety with all other workers as shared knowledge makes for a safer working environment.

■ Follow the workplace policies for your job. Ensure that you know what they are.

Health, Safety and Welfare Regulations Applicable to the Beauty Therapist

The Workplace (Health, Safety and Welfare) Regulations 1992

This regulation covers health, safety and welfare in the workplace.

Workplace means any place where people are employed or are self-employed, it includes the outdoor areas such as paths, etc.

Health issues under this act

Adequate ventilation
Premises must be well ventilated, removing stale air and drawing in fresh clean air without draughts.

Comfortable working temperature
It is difficult to select a temperature to suit everybody, so around 16°C is recommended. The temperature should be comfortable for working but also warm enough for the client who will usually be inactive and may feel cold.

Adequate lighting
Lighting must be adequate to enable people to work and move around safely. It should be suitable for the treatment in progress and where low soft lighting is desirable it must be bright enough to see the machine controls clearly and to operate safely.

Cleanliness and hygiene
Premises must be cleaned regularly to the highest standard. Floors, walls and ceilings together with furniture and fittings should be washed and disinfected where possible. All towels and sheets used should be boil-washed after each client.

Hygiene is discussed more fully in the next chapter.

Waste
Waste must be stored in suitable, covered bins and disposed of in accordance with regulations. Disposable needles must be placed in a 'sharps' box' for collection.

Adequate space for working
Cubicles containing a couch trolley, chair, stool and waste bin should be large enough for the therapist and client to move around easily. There should be adequate space for all staff to move around easily in the salon without having to negotiate obstacles.

Safety issues under this act

Maintenance of equipment
Everything in the workplace, the equipment and systems, should be maintained in efficient working order. If a fault occurs in any machine or other equipment, it must be taken out of use immediately. It must be clearly labelled 'FAULTY, OUT OF USE' and stored away from the working area. The fault must be reported and the appropriate action taken to repair it.

Floors and traffic routes
Floors should be sound and even, with a non-slippery surface and must be kept

free of obstacles. Any spillages such as water, oil, powder, etc., should be wiped up immediately because it will make the floor slippery which may result in someone slipping and falling. Doors should be wide enough for easy access and exit, stairs should be sound and well lit. A handrail should be provided on at least one side of the stairs.

Falls and falling objects

Every effort must be made to prevent anyone falling on the premises. Sound, even, non-slip floors will help. Leads should not trail across the floor but should lie along the wall; stools and bins should be stored under couches; other equipment must not be left around but must be stored correctly.

Every effort must be made to prevent objects falling and injuring people. Storage shelves must be checked regularly and examined for any damage which may weaken them. Objects should be stored and stacked safely in such a way that they are not likely to fall. Shelves should not be overloaded and should have maximum load notices.

Windows

These should be clean and open easily. Ensure that people cannot walk into them if they are open.

Welfare issues under this act

Sanitary conveniences

Toilets and washing facilities should be available to all persons. These rooms should be clean (cleaned and disinfected regularly), well lit and ventilated. There should be hot and cold running water, soap (preferably in a dispenser), and drying facilities such as paper towels or dry air machines (to prevent the spread of micro-organisms).

Drinking water

An adequate supply of fresh drinking water must be provided, either direct mains water, from a chilled water dispenser or bottled water.

Changing rooms

These rooms must be clean, suitable and secure, where outer garments are removed and uniforms put on. Changing rooms are also desirable for clients although the cubicles may also be used if privacy for the user can be ensured.

Facilities for resting and eating

Food and drink should not be consumed in the treatment cubicles or in the salon. A clean room should be allocated for eating. Adequate comfortable chairs should be provided as well as a table or tables on which to place food and drink.

Safety considerations when dealing with hazardous substances

The Control of Substances Hazardous to Health Act 2002 (COSHH)

This law requires employers to control exposure to hazardous substances to prevent ill health. It protects everyone in the workplace from exposure to hazardous substances. Hazardous substances found in the salon include:

- cleaning agents
- disinfectants
- massage products – oils, creams, lotions and talcum powder
- powders or dust

- micro-organisms (i.e. bacteria, viruses, fungi, protozoa)
- parasites
- ozone.

Hazardous substances can enter the body via many routes:

- through broken or damaged skin
- through eyes and ears
- through nose and mouth
- through hair follicles.

Substances hazardous to health may cause the following:

- skin burn
- skin allergic reaction such as dermatitis
- skin irritation
- irritation of nasal passages and lungs or allergies to products, especially fine powder or dust resulting in the development of asthma
- breathing difficulties and respiratory problems, especially dry heat and ozone
- nausea and vomiting if swallowed
- eye damage.

COSHH requires you to:

1 **Assess** the risk from exposure to hazardous substances to anyone using your workplace. You will need to examine all the substances stored and used in your salon and identify the ones that could cause damage or injury. You will need to consider any risks that these substances present to people's health.

2 **Decide** what precautions need to be taken. Check the manufacturers' advice on use, storage and disposal. Read the label carefully. Consider whether the substance can enter the body or damage any part of the body. Take action to protect employees and others.

3 **Wear gloves, masks and other protective clothing** when dealing with hazardous substances. Ensure that your control systems are in place and effective.

4 **Control** or reduce the exposure to hazardous substances. Consider the use of other safer products. Store all products safely and label them clearly to reduce any errors in handling. Buy small quantities of stock and use by their use by date. Take care when handling fine powders such as talcum powder: avoid releasing the fine particles into the air and avoid inhaling any powders, also protect your client. Use small quantities and avoid wastage.

5 **Ensure** that control measures are in place and regularly monitored for effectiveness. Keep records of all control measures and any tests or problems arising. These records should be kept for at least five years.

6 **Prepare** procedures to deal with accidents, incidents and emergencies. Immediate steps must be taken to minimize the harmful effects and damage. These procedures should be clearly written and placed in a prominent and accessible place.

7 **Train** and supervise all staff. Ensure that all employees understand the risks from all the hazardous substances they have to deal with. Inform them of the rules and regulations for using, storing and transporting or disposing of hazardous substances.

8 **Ensure** that all employees understand the importance of reporting any problems or shortcomings when dealing with hazardous substances.

Precautions and responsibilities when dealing with hazardous substances

1 Consider any hazardous substances in your workplace. For the therapist these will include any fine powders, such as face powder or talcum powder, oils, creams or lotions, cleaning agents, sterilizing agents, bacteria, blood.

2 Read the labels and manufacturers' instructions on all the products that you use. Manufacturers are required by law to state the dangers and issue guidelines on storage, use and disposal.

3 Ensure that products are clearly labelled and stored correctly and safely.

4 Ensure that the highest standards of hygiene are implemented to prevent cross infection (this is dealt with in Chapter 2).

5 Avoid blood contamination. Cover any broken skin with a plaster and wear gloves.

6 Ensure the safe disposal of 'sharps' into a 'sharps' box' and dispose of in accordance with the correct procedure.

Safety considerations when using electrical equipment

The Provision and Use of Work Equipment Regulation 1998

The Electricity at Work Regulation 1989

These regulations require that all equipment provided for use at work is:

- suitable and safe for the intended use
- inspected regularly by a competent person and maintained in a safe condition
- used only by therapists who are fully informed, trained and competent in their use.

Therapists use many different types of electrical equipment to treat their clients. It is therefore very important that you understand, and are able to assess, the hazards and risks associated with their use and know what action to take to eliminate or minimize them. The main hazards and risks are:

H exposed parts of the leads, wiring or cables

R contact with these will result in shock or/and burns which may prove fatal

H faulty equipment

R contact will cause electric shock

H faults in the wiring or overloading the circuit

R may cause fires resulting in injury or even death if the fire is severe

H water in the area where electrical equipment is used or working with wet hands

R electric shock

H trailing leads and cables across the floor

R tripping people up and causing injury

H loose fitting bulbs

R falling on clients causing burns or falling on bedding and towels causing fires

H positioning lamps directly over clients

R falling or exploding bulbs may cause burns and injure the client.

Precautions and responsibilities when using electrical equipment

- Annual testing of electrical equipment is required by law.
- Ensure that people using electrical equipment are trained and competent to do so.
- Follow the correct procedures when using electrical equipment.
- Purchase equipment from a reputable dealer who will provide an after sales service.
- Ensure that all equipment is regularly maintained and in a safe condition for use.

- Examine leads and cables regularly to ensure that they are without splits or breaks which may expose bare wires.
- Use proper connectors to join wire and flexes, do not use insulating tape.
- Examine all connections making sure that they are secure.
- Ensure that the cable is firmly clamped into the plug to ensure that the wires, particularly the earth wire, cannot be pulled out of the terminals.
- Do not overload the circuit by using multiple adaptors. If you find others overloading the circuit, explain to them that this is dangerous practice.
- Plug the machine into a near and accessible identified socket so that it can be switched off or disconnected easily in an emergency.
- Keep electrical equipment away from water; do not touch any electrical part with wet hands.
- Ensure that flexes and cables do not trail over the working area; fix them along the wall.
- Examine all equipment regularly, especially portable machines as they are subjected to wear and tear.
- Remove faulty equipment from the working area, label clearly 'FAULTY, DO NOT USE', and inform others that it is faulty.
- Keep a dated record of when checks were carried out, including all findings and maintenance.

Electric Shock

Mild electric shock may be caused by a sudden surge of current. This feels like a sudden tingle and although unpleasant is rarely serious. The main causes are:

- the intensity controls are not at zero when the machine is switched on
- the terminals are pushed into the sockets when the intensity is turned up
- the pads are moved with the intensity turned up
- the intensity control is turned up and down too quickly
- the current discharges through a metal contact.

However, severe electric shock can occur through accidental contact with exposed parts of electrical equipment, appliances and wires.

Direct contact with an electrical current can be fatal.

Definition
An **electric shock** is an injury to the body when a person is exposed to an electric current.

An electric current can pass easily through the body because the body is a good conductor of electricity. There are three main ways in which the body sustains injury:

a. Cardiac arrest due to the effect of the current on the heart.

b. Muscle and tissue destruction as the current passes through the body.

c. Thermal burns of the tissues from contact with the current.

The **symptoms** may include: skin burns, weakness, muscle pain and contraction, heart arrhythmias, cardiac arrest, respiratory failure and unconsciousness.

Action
It is vitally important to act quickly. **Do not** touch the person, ensure that you are safe, then if possible, switch off the source of electricity at the socket switch. Call for help. If the current cannot be turned off, use a wooden broom or chair to push the victim away from the source of the current. **Do not use a wet or metal object.** Check the person's airway, breathing and pulse. Stay with the person until the first aider arrives.

Reporting Health and Safety Issues

Reporting of Injuries, Diseases and Dangerous Occurrences Regulations 1985 (RIDDOR)

This regulation places a legal duty on employers, the self-employed and those in control of premises to report work-related incidents. These incidents must be reported to the Health and Safety Executive (HSE) or your Local Authority (LA).

If you inform the Incident Contact Centre (ICC), they will report and forward the information to the correct enforcing authority on your behalf.

> The Incident Contact Centre (ICC)
> Caerphilly Business Park
> Caerphilly
> CF83 3GG
> Tel: 0845 300 9923
> Internet: www.riddor.gov.uk
> Email: riddor@natbrit.com
> Fax: 0845 300 9924

By law the following incidents must be reported:

- death

- major injuries or poisoning.

- any accident where the person injured is away from work for more than three days

- injuries where members of the public are taken to hospital

- diseases contracted at work

- dangerous occurrences which did not result in reportable injury but may have done.

First Aid at Work

The Health and Safety (First Aid) Regulations 1981

These regulations require all employers to provide adequate and appropriate equipment, facilities and personnel to enable first aid to be given to employees and others if they are injured or become ill at work.

First aid is the immediate treatment administered when any person suffers an injury or becomes ill at work.

The minimum first aid provision at any work place includes:

- a suitably stocked first aid box placed in a precise, easily accessible and clearly labelled site

- an appointed person to take charge of first aid arrangements.

First aid provision must be available at all times to people at work. It may therefore be necessary to train more than one person to be in charge.

The duties of the appointed first aid person will include:

- Taking charge and administering appropriate treatment (providing that they have been trained to do so) when someone is injured or falls ill.

- Calling an ambulance if required, depending on the seriousness of the injury.

- Taking responsibility for the contents of the first aid box and restocking as required.

The designated first aid person must have received training in administering first aid and hold a current first aid certificate. Appointed persons should not give first aid for which they have not been trained.

Short emergency first aid training courses are available. This training must have the approval of the HSE.

All employees must be informed of the first aid arrangements. Notices situated in clearly visible places must inform them of who and where the first aid appointed persons are and where the first aid box is located.

Figure 1.1   First aid box

Manual Handling

The Manual Handling Operations Regulations 1992

This regulation requires all employers to assess the risk to employees when lifting or handling heavy goods and to provide training in safe techniques.

More than a third of all over three-day injuries reported each year to the HSE and LAs are caused by manual handling, i.e. lifting, transporting or supporting loads by hand or bodily force. The accidents primarily result in back injuries, but hands, arms and feet may also be injured. These injuries may build up over time as a result of repetitive movements or may be caused by single poor lifting techniques or too heavy a load. As a therapist you may be required to receive, check and handle deliveries and transport these to the stock room or move couches in the salon. It is therefore essential that you are able to assess the risk and protect yourself from injury.

Before lifting or moving anything assess the risk:

- How heavy is the load?
- Can you reduce the load?
- Do you have to lift it off the floor? (This produces the greatest risk.)
- Can you get assistance from another person?
- How far do you have to move it?
- Can you rest it half way on a chair or table to ease the effort?

Lifting techniques

1   Feet apart on either side of the load for a balanced stable base

2   Good posture, maintain natural curves

Figure 1.2   Feet on either side of the load for a stable base

Figure 1.4   Take a firm grip and hold the load close to the body

Figure 1.3   Bend the knees and keep the arms into the sides

3   Tuck chin in, keep a straight back, lower and bend the knees

4   Take a firm grip

5   Keep the arms in to the sides, hold the load close to the body. If you hold it away from the body this increases the leverage and increases the risk of injury

6   Lift smoothly, do not jerk or twist the body as you lift. Move the feet and place the load in position

7   Do not twist the trunk when placing the load down.

Figure 1.5   Lift smoothly. Do not twist the trunk when placing the load down

Protect your back

Back strains and injuries can also occur as a result of incorrect posture and stance. When performing treatments, ensure that you adopt the correct position. Place the machine on your dominant side to avoid reaching over the client when adjusting the terminals. Sit with your weight evenly distributed and your feet apart, keep the back straight, do not twist your body as

you work and avoid stretching over the client.

Fire Precautions

The Fire Precautions (Workplace) Regulations 1997

These regulations require the employer to ensure that safety measures are in place to prevent and deal with the outbreak of fire in the salon. The employer must assess the fire risks, keep a written record of these risks and inform all employees of the findings. The following precautions and measures must be in place:

- Smoke alarms or other fire detection equipment must be fitted, checked regularly and maintained in working good order.
- Fire fighting equipment must be in good working order and suitable for the type of fire.
- Fire fighting equipment must be clearly visible and easily accessible.
- Fire doors should be fitted if the risk of fire is assessed as high.
- A means of escape must be provided and marked 'fire exit'.
- Doors should be left unlocked and kept free of obstruction for quick escape.
- All employees must be kept informed and trained in fire procedures.
- Notices for fire procedures and evacuation should be clear and prominently displayed.

Fire is a hazard in any place of work and it is very important that you familiarize yourself with your salon's fire procedures and evacuation drill. If a fire occurs you will need to act very quickly, it is therefore very important to know exactly what to do to ensure your own safety and the safety of others. Remember, others may panic and so it is important that you stay calm and take control of the situation. Knowing exactly what procedure to take beforehand will enable you to act promptly.

All members of staff should ensure that they receive training in fire drill and fire evacuation procedures.

Fire evacuation procedures must be practised regularly.

All staff should know:

- How to recognize the sound of the fire or smoke alarms.
- Whom to report to and how to raise the alarm.
- How to contact the emergency services or inform the person who is responsible for doing this.
- The exact position of the fire fighting equipment and how to use it should the fire be small and easy to control.
- The colour coding on the fire extinguishers in your salon and what type

of fire they are suitable for (these are not included in this text as they may change in the future, but ensure that you check all those in your salon). Read the instructions on each one and if you are unsure of any detail, ask the supervisor or the person responsible.

- Where the exit doors and exit routes are and in what order the salon is to be evacuated.
- What and how checks are to be made on the numbers of staff and clients or others to ensure that everyone is safe.
- How you may contain the fire and limit the damage, for example by closing

any doors other than exit doors, closing windows, switching off electrical equipment, using a fire blanket to smother the fire. These actions must only be taken if it is safe to do so and would not put yourself or anyone else at risk.

Identify anything that may be a fire hazard in your workplace and take every precaution to avoid risk to yourself and others.

Draw a plan of the position of all the fire fighting equipment in your workplace. Label each piece, state its colour coding and the type of fire it is suitable for.

Risk Assessment

You may be required to carry out a risk assessment in your workplace to ensure that everything possible is in place to prevent anyone being harmed or contracting illness. It is a legal requirement to keep a written record of the risk assessment if there are five or more employees but it is good practice to do so anyway. You must be able to identify hazards, risks and aspects in your workplace that could cause harm to yourself or others. Consider the following: safe maintenance, care and use of equipment; the safe use, handling and storage of hazardous substances; safe and hygienic working practices; personal and salon hygiene; adequate procedures for dealing with emergencies such as fire, shock, etc.; proper environmental and welfare requirements.

Procedure

Walk around your salon, looking for all the hazards which pose a risk of harm to

anyone entering the salon. Consider the hazards mentioned in this text or any others. Ask colleagues if they have identified anything that may pose a risk to anyone. Write a list of all the hazards that you have identified.

Check the procedures and controls already in place and ensure that they meet legal requirements. List the hazards and risks that require action and state the action needed to eliminate these risks. Give priority to high risks, those that may cause the most serious damage and those that affect the greatest number of people. These should receive immediate attention. Inform all staff of your findings and ensure that they are trained in the new procedures. Set a date for the next risk assessment.

Keep a record of the risk assessment in an easily accessible identified place.

Examples of risks in a salon

High risk
Unsafe equipment, uneven and cluttered floor space
Electrical equipment (units, cables, sockets, leads, plugs)

Substances and materials
Unhygienic practices
Unsafe behaviour
Unsafe storage
Unsafe practices

Low risk
Spillages
Breakages
Environmental factors

Example record card for risk assessment

Name of workplace: Signed: ....
....   Date: ....

List the significant hazards	List the groups of people who are at risk	List the existing controls or note where they can be found	List and date the actions to be taken to introduce effective controls

Local Authority Regulations

The Local Government (Miscellaneous Provisions) Act 1982

Local authorities issue licences and register businesses offering beauty therapy treatments including massage. They also issue regulations which, by law, you must comply with. Before setting up a business you must contact your local authority to ensure that you comply with the exact requirements. When you meet all the requirements you will be given with a certificate of registration. These by-laws are mainly concerned with matters of hygiene and safety as explained in this text. Environmental Health Officers have the right under this law to inspect your business and can issue fines or withdraw your registration if you are not complying with the regulations.

Contact your local authority and ask for the regulations relating to setting up a business offering beauty treatments.

QUESTIONS

1 Briefly explain the role of the health and safety inspectorate.

2 List the working practices involved in your job that could cause harm to yourself or others.

3 Identify potential hazards and risks in your workplace that could cause harm to yourself and others.

4 Explain why the use of electrical equipment could pose a high risk to yourself and others.

5 List five precautions you would take to protect yourself and others from injury when carrying out electrical treatments.

6 Give the procedure you would follow if you had identified a hazard but you were not able to deal with yourself.

7 List five substances or products which could pose a risk in your workplace.

8 Explain the importance of maintaining good posture and adopting accurate lifting techniques in the workplace.

9 Discuss the environmental factors that contribute to health and safety in the workplace.

10 Give the name and location of the person responsible for health and safety in your workplace.

2 Hygiene

OBJECTIVES

After you have studied this chapter you will be able to:

1 Distinguish between infection and infestation.

2 Differentiate between bacteria, viruses, fungi and protozoa.

3 List some common diseases caused by each micro-organism.

4 Distinguish between natural immunity and artificial immunity.

5 List the ways in which micro-organisms enter the body.

6 Explain how micro-organisms may be transmitted.

7 List the required conditions for the growth of bacteria.

8 Describe the cause, symptoms and transmission of hepatitis.

9 Describe the cause, symptoms and transmission of HIV which causes AIDS.

10 Distinguish between ectoparasites and endoparasites.

11 Explain the meaning and terminology used in control of micro-organisms.

12 List three methods of sterilization.

13 Select methods of sterilization for use in the salon.

14 List a selection of disinfectants available.

15 Select appropriate disinfectants for specific apparatus.

16 Discuss the factors to be considered in maintaining high standards of salon hygiene.

17 Discuss the factors to be considered in maintaining high standards of personal hygiene.

18 Describe the factors to be considered when setting up a salon.

Hygiene deals with the precautions and procedures necessary for maintaining health and preventing the spread of disease. In the salon, the highest priority must be given to preventing infection, cross infection and infestation. The beauty therapist carries a heavy responsibility for protecting herself, other staff and the clients from the risk of contamination by micro-organisms which cause disease.

Figure 2.1   a) Bed with easy-clean cover; b) Heavy duty trolley

Infection, Cross Infection and Infestation

Infection

An infection or infectious disease is caused by micro-organisms invading the body. The symptoms and severity of the illness will depend on the type of invading micro-organism and the part of the body affected.

Infestation

An infestation is the invasion of the body by animal parasites, such as lice, worms and flukes; they may live in or on the body. Some parasites merely cause itchy irritation, while others cause serious illness.

Micro-organisms or microbes

There are many different types of micro-organisms present in the environment. The main groups include:

- bacteria
- viruses
- fungi, yeasts
- protozoa.

Micro-organisms entering the body do not always produce disease as the immune system is stimulated to protect the body. However if the invading organisms are in large enough numbers to overcome the immune system then disease and illness will occur. Disease will also occur if the body has little immunity to the invading microbe or if the immune system has itself been damaged by disease as in AIDS. If the body's defences are overcome then the microbes will cause damage or destruction of the cells. Some microbes release toxins which destroy the cells, while others multiply and directly destroy them. The various micro-organisms produce a wide variety of diseases, each one showing particular symptoms. When the immune system fails to contain a disease, drugs are necessary to treat the infections. Antibacterial or antibiotic drugs are used to treat bacterial infections. Antiviral drugs are used to treat viral infections, antifungal drugs to treat fungal and yeast infections and antiprotozoal to treat infections by protozoa.

Ways in which the body resists infection

Non-specific resistance

1   Unbroken skin forms a physical barrier.
2   Mucous membranes, mucus, hairs and cilia help to trap and filter microbes.
3   Saliva washes microbes from teeth and mouth.
4   Tears wash microbes from the eyes.
5   Urine washes microbes from the urethra.
6   Faeces remove microbes from the bowel.
7   The acidic pH of the skin limits growth of bacteria.

8   Sebum produces an oily film which protects the skin.
9   Gastric juices destroy bacteria in the stomach.
10   Various antimicrobial substances are produced by the body in response to infection (e.g. interferon).
11   Macrophages and granulocytes ingest and destroy micro-organisms by a process of phagocytosis.

Specific resistance (immunity)

The body also produces specific antibodies to destroy a particular antigen. This specific resistance to disease is known as **immunity**. Disease will occur if the body has little immunity to the invading microbes, or if the immune system has itself been damaged, as happens with the Human Immunodeficiency Virus (HIV). Immunity is gained as a result of the body coming into contact with an antigen and producing T cells or antibodies to control it. Immunity may be acquired naturally or artificially.

Natural active immunity
This is obtained when a person comes into contact with a particular microbe and produces antibodies or T cells to repel and control it. These antibodies remain in the body to control future infection. Many infectious diseases occur only once in a lifetime as immunity is lifelong while others may recur as immunity may last for only a few years.

Natural passive immunity
This involves the transfer of antibodies from an immunized donor to a recipient. Immunity may be passed from mother to baby via the placenta or mother's milk.

Artificial active immunity

Artificial immunity can be provided by the use of vaccines. These are prepared from altered or diluted forms of the organism. Once they are introduced into the body, they stimulate the immune system in the same way as an infection, but are not strong enough to cause the disease.

Artificial passive immunity

Another type of immunization relies on transferring antibodies from someone who has recovered from that particular disease. The transfer is made via a serum containing the antibodies.

Invasion

Micro-organisms enter the body via many routes:

1. Through broken or damaged skin.
2. Through orifices, such as the nose, mouth, anus, vagina and urethra.
3. Through the eyes and ears.
4. Into hair follicles.
5. Into the blood stream via bloodsucking insects such as mosquitoes and lice.

Some micro-organisms produce immediate symptoms, while others can lie dormant for a long time and attack when the body's immune system is low.

Transmission

Micro-organisms are transmitted in many ways:

1. By droplet infection: an infected person coughing and sneezing or spitting will expel organisms into the air where they may be inhaled by others.
2. By handling contaminated articles, such as clothing, towels and equipment, when micro-organisms may be transmitted to the handler.
3. Dirty surfaces or dusty atmospheres will contain micro-organisms, which may be inhaled or may enter via the eyes or ears.
4. Organisms present in faeces and urine may be transferred to others if the hands are not thoroughly washed after visiting the toilet.
5. Food may become contaminated by handling with unwashed hands and also by flies carrying contamination from excreta and rubbish. Water may become contaminated and then organisms will be transmitted to humans through drinking the water or eating foods washed with it.
6. Through contact with animals.
7. Through direct contact with others, for example kissing, hand contact or touching.
8. Organisms may be spread through intermediary hosts, such as fleas and bloodsucking insects.
9. Sexual intercourse can spread certain organisms which produce diseases.
10. Contaminated blood, if transmitted to another person, can cause serious and, sometimes, fatal illness. Organisms can be transmitted through blood transfusion, infected needles or at any time when the blood of the carrier (infected person) enters the body of the recipient.

Hepatitis B and HIV are transmitted in this way, and great care must be taken in the salon to avoid any contact with blood. Needles and ear piercing equipment must be carefully disposed of into sharps' boxes. Any blood spots should be dealt with by wearing gloves and using strong disinfectant (e.g. household bleach).

11 Infection can be caused by the spread of certain organisms within one's own body. These organisms may be harmless in one part of the body, but will produce inflammation in another, for example certain organisms in the intestine are harmless, but if they invade the bladder they produce cystitis.

The conditions required for the growth of micro-organisms are:

1 A food supply.

2 A water supply or moisture.

3 Warmth, pathogenic bacteria favour body temperature of 37°C. Low temperatures found in the refrigerator or freezer will prevent growth of bacteria but will not destroy them.

4 Dark conditions, strong UVL will kill bacteria.

5 Oxygen is required by some bacteria for aerobic respiration but others are anaerobic and survive without oxygen.

6 Slightly alkaline conditions. (The acidity of the skin's acid mantle, helps to protect against growth of bacteria.)

Bacteria

Bacteria are single-cell organisms varying in size from 0.2 to 2.0 μm in diameter. They are found everywhere in the environment and can be seen through an optical microscope. Many bacteria are harmless and useful to man and are called **non-pathogenic bacteria.** Some are used in the production of food, such as cheese and yoghurt. Others help to dispose of unwanted organic material, such as the breakdown of sewage, rendering it harmless. Some bacteria in the human intestine help to synthesise vitamins K and B_2.

The harmful bacteria which cause disease are known as **pathogenic bacteria** or **pathogens**. Bacteria are the simplest

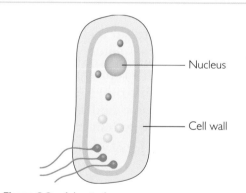

Figure 2.2   A bacterium

of living organisms, composed of a single cell with cytoplasm surrounded by a protective cell membrane but devoid of organelles. They multiply rapidly by dividing into two, known as **binary fission**. This can occur every 20 minutes and a single bacterium may give rise to 16 million bacteria per day. Some bacteria have whip-like projections on the surface of the cell called flagella which enable the bacteria to move around. Bacteria may be aerobic, requiring oxygen to sustain life, or they may be anaerobic, able to survive without oxygen.

The aerobic variety is found invading surface tissues of the skin and mucous membranes of the respiratory tract. The anaerobic variety is found in the bowel or deep wounds. Some bacteria develop into spores; these can lie dormant for long periods of time and become active when conditions are suitable. Spores develop a hard, thick outer shell which protects the contents and makes them very difficult to destroy. They are more resistant to heat and disinfectants. Higher temperatures and strong chemical disinfectants are required to kill spores.

Types of bacteria

Bacteria are classified according to their shape:

- cocci are spherical
- bacilli are rod-shaped
- spirochetes are spirals or curves.

Cocci

These spherical-shaped bacteria may form clusters known as staphylococci, or they may form chains known as streptococci or they may form pairs known as diplococci. They can cause a wide variety of conditions, such as boils, carbuncles, impetigo, sore throat, meningitis and pneumonia.

Bacilli

These rod-shaped bacteria cause serious illness, such as diptheria, tuberculosis and typhoid fever.

Spirochetes

These spiral- or curved-shaped bacteria include spirillium and vibros and cause venereal disease, such as syphilis, and serious disease, such as cholera.

Bacteria cause disease by producing toxins or poisons which are harmful to body cells. The body protects itself against bacterial infection by several methods:

1 By producing antitoxins which neutralize toxins produced by the bacteria.

2 By producing large numbers of white cells, macrophages and granulocytes, which circulate in the blood and which engulf and destroy bacteria.

3 By producing antibodies which attack and destroy the bacteria.

Cocci (spherical)   Bacilli (rod-shaped)   Spirochete (spirals)

Figure 2.3   Types of bacteria

The discovery of penicillin and the development of other antibiotics and antibacterials means that bacterial infections can be brought under control. Antibiotics must be used in adequate doses for at least 5 days. Some antibiotics kill the bacteria directly, while others prevent multiplication of the bacteria.

Bacteria grow and multiply if the conditions are right. These are:

1 A food supply.

2 A water supply or moisture.

3 Warmth; pathogenic bacteria favour a body temperature of 37 °C. Low temperatures found in the refrigerator or freezer will limit the growth of bacteria, but will not destroy them.

4 Dark conditions; strong ultraviolet light will kill bacteria.

5 Oxygen is required by some bacteria for aerobic respiration, but others are anaerobic and survive without oxygen.

6 Slightly alkaline conditions. The acidity of the skin (acid mantle), helps to protect against the growth of bacteria.

Viruses

Viruses are the smallest known infective particles; smaller than bacteria, they can only be seen through an electron microscope. They are between 0.1 and 0.2 μm in size and they vary in shape from spheres, cubes or rods.

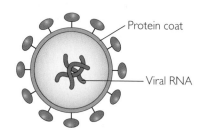

Figure 2.4   A virus

They consist of a core of nucleic acid, RNA or DNA, enclosed in a protein shell or capsid. Viruses cannot metabolize or reproduce; they are parasitic, living inside a host cell. Once inside, a virus causes the host cell to replicate, that is make copies of the virus. After the virus enters the host cell there is a period of 'incubation' – the host cells show no sign of disease. Eventually, the host cell is destroyed and hundreds of new viruses are released which attack other cells. Many cycles of viral spread occur and more and more host cells are affected; eventually typical signs and symptoms of the disease occur. By the time the symptoms appear, the viruses are so numerous that antiviral drugs have limited effect. The body protects itself against viral infection by producing specific antibodies. These will also provide future immunity to some diseases; immunity can be produced artificially to combat some viral infections. Body cells also produce 'interferons' which interfere with the multiplication of viruses.

Antiviral drugs are now available; some prevent the multiplication of viruses while others alter the DNA within the cell, preventing the virus from using it. In this way, the spread of infection is halted. Viral diseases include the common cold, influenza, poliomyelitis, mumps, herpes simplex and zoster, chickenpox, warts, hepatitis and HIV.

Hepatitis and HIV

The two most serious viral infections that could be transmitted between clients or staff and clients in the salon are hepatitis B and HIV, both of which are carried in the blood. Minute amounts of blood or organic material can carry infection, it may not be visible to the naked eye. The correct hygiene procedures must be followed to prevent any possibility of infection (see page 32).

Hepatitis – inflammation of the liver

Hepatitis is caused by viruses or by amoebae. There are many forms of the disease, each having similar symptoms but contracted by different viruses, namely: hepatitis A virus, hepatitis B virus and hepatitis non-A and -B.

Symptoms of hepatitis
1 Fever.
2 Loss of appetite.
3 Nausea and vomiting.
4 Jaundice (yellow colouring of the skin and whites of the eyes).
5 Pain in the abdomen with tenderness over the liver.
6 Dark urine.

Patients feel very ill for several months and need a long period of convalescence. Patients recover eventually but death may result; death rarely occurs with hepatitis A but is more common with hepatitis B.

Hepatitis A virus
Hepatitis A virus has a short incubation period of around three weeks. It is contracted through faecal contact due to poor sanitation and poor personal hygiene. It may be contracted by UK residents travelling abroad where faecal–oral contamination is likely and waste disposal may be basic with open sewers, etc. The virus may have already been passed on before the sufferer realizes that she is infected as it is most contagious during the incubation period. It does not cause any lasting damage to the liver.

Hepatitis B virus
This has a long incubation period of around three months. It is transmitted through breaks in the skin or by punctures with contaminated equipment. It may also be transmitted sexually or following transfusion with contaminated blood. Highly infectious mothers usually pass it on to their babies. The virus is detected in blood, saliva, semen and body fluids. High-risk groups are: drug abusers, homosexuals and renal dialysis patients.

The disease is most contagious during the incubation period when a carrier may not be showing any symptoms. There are thousands of symptomless carriers worldwide. Hepatitis B can cause lasting chronic liver damage that may result in death.

The particular danger to the beauty therapist and her clients is the transmission of this disease during electrolysis, or on any occasion where blood contamination is likely. Blood, tissue fluid and skin debris may be carried on the needle and transmitted from one client to another or to the therapist by accidental needle stabs.

Disposable 'sterex' needles must always be used in the salon to prevent the spread of this disease. Used needles should be very carefully handled and disposed of in a sharps' box, which must be incinerated. Hepatitis B is a particularly resistant virus. Sterilization using the autoclave and the use of disinfectants, such as 70 per cent isopropyl alcohol and chlorine, are the most effective methods of control.

Hepatitis non-A and non-B

These have an incubation period of around one month and are distinct from the previous two but produce very similar symptoms. They may be contracted from contaminated food and water or blood transfusions. They can cause inflammation of the liver followed by cirrhosis (scarring of the liver).

Human Immunodeficiency Virus (HIV) which causes Aids – Acquired Immune Deficiency Syndrome

Aids was first reported in the New England Medical Journal in 1981 and by the end of that year the first case was reported in the United Kingdom. It is a disease which affects both homosexuals and heterosexuals and both males and females.

In 1983 scientists in the United States of America and France isolated the HIV virus which causes Aids. This virus attacks a group of cells called T4 or the T helper cells which play a part in coordinating the action of the immune system.

Following infection with HIV, there may be no immediate symptoms and the incubation period may be up to eight years. There are many thousands of symptomless carriers worldwide. The first symptoms are usually fatigue, fever, swollen glands and headaches. After a few weeks these symptoms may disappear.

Some time later the next stage of the disease appears when the glands of the neck, armpit and groin become chronically swollen. During this time the helper T cells which play a key role in antibody production, diminish in number until eventually the body's immune system is destroyed. The body is then defenceless against a wide variety of diseases which include pneumonia, tuberculosis, thrush and Karposi's sarcoma (a deadly skin cancer which produces purple-brownish marks on the skin). The heart, liver and brain may also become affected, leading to dementia and death.

This virus has been located in blood, semen, vaginal fluid, tears, saliva and cerebro-spinal fluid. However, to be transmitted the virus must be present in large numbers and these are found only in blood, semen and vaginal secretions.

Ways in which HIV is transmitted:

1 Sexual intercourse with an infected person male to male, male to female or female to male.

2 Through blood exchange from open bleeding cuts and wounds; from contaminated needles or other contaminated instruments piercing the skin.

3 Infected mothers pass it to their babies through the placenta,

during birth or through breast feeding.

No cure has been found to date and preventative measures must be taken to avoid spread of the disease. The virus is quite fragile outside the body and can be destroyed by: autoclaving all contaminated instruments; washing towels, dishes etc. at 56°C for 10 minutes; cleaning surfaces with 70 per cent alcohol or chlorine bleach; and by soaking blood spills with chlorine bleach for ten minutes.

Fungi

Fungi are larger than bacteria; they may be unicellular, as in yeasts, or multicellular, as in moulds. The cells contain nuclei and other cell components, but do not contain chlorophyll. They obtain their food by secreting enzymes through the cell walls. This digests any organic matter which is then absorbed as liquid food. Fungi may be saprophytes which obtain food from dead organic matter, or parasites, living off plants, animals or humans and feeding off skin and mucous membranes and producing diseases. They reproduce by forming spores. The unicellular fungi and spores are not visible to the naked eye, but the filamentous fungi forming mycelia are visible, for example moulds and mildews.

Fungi require similar conditions to bacteria for growth, i.e.:

- a food supply
- damp, moist conditions
- warmth
- oxygen, although some survive for a short time without.

Diseases caused by fungi are:

1 Ringworm:
   (a) Of the foot: *Tinea pedis* (athlete's foot).
   (b) Of the body: *Tinea corporis*.
   (c) Of the head: *Tinea capitis*.
   (d) Of the nail: *Tinea unguium*.
2 Thrush, which is caused by the fungus *Candida albicans*.
3 More serious internal fungal infections of the lungs and heart can be fatal.

Once fungal infections invade the body and grow, antifungal drugs are required to control the infection as the condition will rarely improve without drugs. Some antifungal drugs are applied to the areas, while others are taken by mouth. They destroy the fungal cell wall and the cell dies.

Figure 2.5   Fungi

Protozoa

These are the simplest of single-celled animals, slightly bigger than bacteria. Each protozoa is composed of cytoplasm containing a nucleus and organelles surrounded by a cell wall or membrane. They move around by pushing out pseudopodia. Many types are known to exist as parasites on humans, particularly in the bowel. Some are harmless causing few symptoms, while others cause different types of illness, some very serious depending on the organism involved.

Protozoa may be transmitted from contaminated food and water, through sexual contact and by bites from insects. They may infect the bowel causing diarrhoea with general ill health and malaise, or they may cause serious illness, such as sleeping sickness, malaria and amoebic dysentery.

As protozoa are difficult to eradicate, treatment requires antiprotozoal drugs to be given over a long period of time.

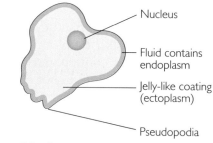

Figure 2.6   Protozoa

- Nucleus
- Fluid contains endoplasm
- Jelly-like coating (ectoplasm)
- Pseudopodia

Animal Parasites

Parasites are living organisms that live in or on another living organism and derive their food supply from that host.

Definitions
Ectoparasites live outside the host (e.g. lice and fleas).
Endoparasites live inside the host (e.g. tapeworms or threadworms, round-worms and flukes).

The presence of any parasite on the body is known as an **infestation**.

Ectoparasites

Head lice (*Pediculus capitis*)
The head louse is an insect found on the human scalp. It obtains its nourishment by piercing the skin and sucking blood. The adult female is slightly larger than the male, about 2–3 mm long and 1 mm wide. The female lays white, shiny oval-shaped eggs called nits; they are cemented to the

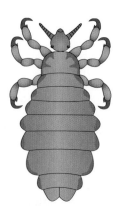

Figure 2.7   Head louse

hair close to the scalp. They take approximately one week to mature and can reproduce in another week. The life cycle of a louse lasts for 4–5 weeks, during which time the female will lay around 300 eggs. They cause intense itching and secondary infections may result due to scratching. Lice and nits may be killed by special shampoos or lotions containing insecticide and combing out with a fine-tooth comb.

Body lice (*Pediculus corporis*)

These are similar but larger than head lice. They obtain nutrients by sucking blood and laying eggs in underclothing. The crab louse is smaller and is found in pubic and underarm hair. Treatment is by insecticidal shampoo and clothing, towels, etc., that have been in contact with body lice must be washed in insecticidal soap and boil washed.

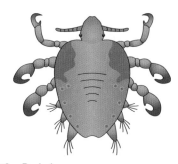

Figure 2.8   Body louse

Itch mites (*Sarcoptes scabiei*)

A tiny animal which burrows into the skin producing a condition called scabies. It has eight legs and is around 0.3 mm long and 0.2 mm wide. The fertilized female burrows into the skin forming dark lines about 1 cm long. She lays around 60 eggs in the burrows which hatch in 4–8 days. The burrows are commonly seen between

Figure 2.9   Itch mite

the fingers, on the front of the wrists, forearms or maybe on male genitalia. They cause intense irritation, vesicles, papules and pustules. They are easily passed from person to person. Medical opinion should be sought and any clothing, towels, etc., that have come into contact with such a client must be burned.

Fleas

The flea is an insect with three pairs of legs which enable it to jump long distances from host to host. It obtains nourishment by biting and sucking the blood of the host. The bites cause red spots usually found in groups; they are intensely itchy. Fleas lay eggs in dust, carpets or furniture. They can be eliminated by spraying with insecticides, washing clothing and bedding and thorough cleaning of soft furnishings. The flea was responsible for carrying the plague.

Figure 2.10   A flea

Endoparasites

These include a variety of worms and flukes. Infestation is usually the result of poor standards of hygiene and insanitary conditions. Worms may be passed on to humans through contaminated food or

Figure 2.11   Worms and flukes

water, while undercooked pork and beef are a source of tapeworms. Threadworms, tapeworms and roundworms live in the intestine and may cause diarrhoea, weakness and anaemia. Liver flukes live in the bile ducts and liver causing jaundice, while some serious types of fluke invade small blood vessels causing serious illness.

The body's defences are not effective against these infestations and drug treatment is essential to eliminate the worms. These anthelmintic drugs kill or paralyse the worms and they pass out of the body in faeces. If serious complications have occurred, other drugs may be necessary to deal with these.

Methods of Controlling Micro-organisms

The process of controlling micro-organisms in the salon is the responsibility of all therapists and must be taken seriously. Correct hygiene procedures must be adopted as a matter of routine. Instruments must always be cleaned after use and then sterilized or disinfected.

Various words are used to explain hygiene procedures. Their meaning must be clearly understood so that the appropriate methods are selected.

Definitions

Antibiotic an organic chemical substance which in dilute solution can destroy or inhibit the growth of bacteria and some other micro-organisms. They are used to treat infectious diseases in humans, animals and plants.

Antiseptic a chemical agent which destroys or inhibits the growth of micro-organisms on living tissues, thus limiting or preventing the harmful results of infection (usually used on wounds, sores or skin cleansing).

Aseptic methods procedures adopted for creating conditions for avoiding infection.

Bactericide a chemical agent which, under defined conditions, is capable of killing bacteria, but not necessarily the spores.

Bacteriostat/fungistat chemical agents which under defined conditions are capable of inhibiting the multiplication of bacteria/fungi.

Biocide, fungicide, virucide, sporicide these words imply the destruction of bacteria, fungi, viruses and spores. Biocides kill everything.

Disinfectant a chemical agent which destroys micro-organisms but not spores (usually used on articles, implements, surfaces, drains, etc.).

Sanitation the establishment of conditions favourable to health and preventing the spread of disease.

Sepsis/septic being infected by bacteria; usually associated with pus formation.

Sterilization the total destruction or removal of all living micro-organisms and their spores.

Sterilization and disinfection

While it is impossible to create a perfectly sterile environment in the salon, every effort must be made to limit the growth and to destroy micro-organisms by practising high standards of hygiene. The clients and therapists must be protected from cross infection.

Most treatments require the therapist to touch the client, therefore every precaution must be taken to prevent cross infection from one to the other. The therapist's hands must be washed using bactericidal lotions and the client's skin must be cleaned by taking a shower or cleansing and toning the face for facial work and wiping over the area with surgical spirit for body treatments. Any small cuts and abrasions on the therapist's hands or on the client's skin must be covered with waterproof plaster. If there is any danger of blood seepage, the treatment should not be carried out.

For some treatments good quality fine surgical gloves could be worn to protect against any contamination. Care must be taken when removing gloves, peel carefully from the open wrist end so that the glove ends up inside out thus containing any contamination.

Extreme care must be taken when practising procedures which pierce the skin. In certain procedures, such as epilation, red vein therapy, etc., it is necessary to pierce the skin, but other procedures may result in blood loss due to accidental piercing of the skin. All blood spills must be dealt with immediately because serious diseases such as HIV and hepatitis can be transmitted via blood contamination.

Disposable needles must be used for treating clients in the salon; a new needle must be used at the commencement of treatment and disposed of after use. They should be carefully removed from the chuck using forceps and placed in a sharps' box. Disposable equipment should always be used if it is economically viable. Reusable equipment should be sterilized if suitable otherwise must be disinfected.

All equipment and instruments contaminated with blood or body fluids must be sterilized or disposed of in sealed plastic containers and incinerated.

Cleaning of equipment

All articles must be thoroughly clean before being sterilized or disinfected. The articles should be thoroughly soaked, washed and scrubbed with a hard brush in water and detergent. Care must be taken to reach the more inaccessible parts so that all matter is removed. Finally, they should be rinsed thoroughly under running water.

This procedure is very important for the following reasons:

1 To remove dirt and all organic matter which may be left on the article.

2 To remove all infective matter.

3 To remove all grease or oil which forms a barrier and interferes with

the sterilizing or disinfecting process, reducing its effectiveness.

4 To remove all dirt and organic matter which would harden, forming a permanent coating on the articles. This would interfere with sterilizing or disinfecting and would cause deterioration of certain instruments.

Sterilization

Sterilization is the best procedure for small instruments and should be a major consideration when purchasing these articles. The therapist should check with the manufacturer that the materials are suitable for the chosen method of sterilization. Instruments made of stainless steel and certain plastics are suitable, although sharp edges may be blunted by exposure to heat.

There are three main methods of sterilization available, but they are not all suitable for use in the salon.

Sterilization by radiation

Two types of rays are used:

1 **Gamma radiation** is only suitable for use on a large scale. Articles to be sterilized are prepacked and exposed to radiation. Colour change indicators are used in the packages to show that sterilization has been achieved. There is little temperature rise and it is, therefore, particularly useful for heat-sensitive materials. Disposable needles are usually sterilized in this way. It has the advantage that materials can be prepacked before sterilization.

Figure 2.12 Germicidal UVL cabinet designed to sanitize but not sterilize

2 **Ultraviolet radiation** is no longer recommended for sterilization. It will destroy bacteria, but spores are resistant. It is also difficult to ensure penetration of the rays and articles require turning to ensure irradiation of all surfaces. Ultraviolet cabinets are frequently found in hair and beauty salons, and although they must not be used as sterilizers, they can be used for storing articles after they have been sterilized.

Sterilization by gas

Two gases are used:

1 Ethylene oxide at a temperature of 20–56 °C.

2 Formaldehyde at a temperature of 70 °C.

These gases are used in chambers into which the articles are placed for a certain period of time. They are not suitable for salon use as they are difficult to handle and can form explosive mixtures with air. However, formaldehyde cabinets are still found in some salons.

Sterilization by heat (suitable for use in salons)

Two methods can be used:

1 Dry heat.

2 Moist heat.

With all methods of heat sterilization, the combination of correct temperature and time of exposure are necessary for sterility to be achieved. For moist heat, the pressure in the sterilizer is also important. The sterilization process can be broken up into four time factors:

1 Heating up time: the time taken for the sterilizer to reach the sterilizing temperature.

2 Heat penetration time: the time taken for all parts of the load to reach the sterilizing temperature.

3 Holding time: this is the time required to sterilize the load at the selected temperature.

4 Safety time: this is an addition of 50 per cent to the holding time to ensure that resistant spores are destroyed.

Both methods are suitable for salon use as small models are manufactured for sterilizing small instruments. Hot air ovens and glass bead sterilizers are used for dry heat sterilization, while pressure vessels called autoclaves are used for moist heat.

The process of boiling in water is no longer considered as a method of sterilization as spores will survive at this temperature. It is now considered to be a process of disinfecting.

Dry heat

Dry heat ovens These ovens are electrically heated with a fan to circulate the air.

A dial thermometer is fitted to indicate the temperature reached within the oven. Dry heat must reach a temperature of 140 °C to kill bacterial spores. However, the higher the temperature, the shorter the exposure time. Therefore, temperatures of 150–180 °C are commonly used. The following temperatures and corresponding timings are issued by the Medical Research Council:

Dry heat temperatures and timings	
Temperature °C	Exposure time in minutes
160	45
170	18
180	7½
190	1½

This covers both holding time and safety time.

Glass bead sterilisers These are suitable for very small articles (read the manufacturer's instructions). They are made of an electrically heated box covered by an insulating case. The box is filled with tiny glass beads. The temperature can range from 190–300 °C, and the sterilizing times will vary accordingly; be sure to follow the instructions on the model.

These have the disadvantages that they are only suitable for small objects (e.g. needles or forceps) and that the objects cannot be fully immersed. Therefore, a small part outside the beads will remain unsterilized.

Figure 2.13   Glass bead sterilizer operates up to 300 °C

Figure 2.14   An automatic electronic autoclave

Moist heat

Autoclave This is a vessel which boils water under pressure so that higher temperatures can be reached. It sterilizes by steam under pressure. Water boils at atmospheric pressure at 100 °C, but if the pressure is increased, then the temperature at which the water boils is raised. The autoclave is a closed vessel which is constructed to withstand high pressure so that the temperature of the water and steam will reach the 100–150 °C needed for sterilization. Air must be eliminated from the vessel in order to achieve the following pressure/temperature relationships.

Pressure temperature relationships for the autoclave	
Pressure in psi (pounds per square inch)	Boiling point °C
10	115
15	121
32	134

For sterilizing with moist heat, the following temperatures and corresponding timings are issued by the Medical Research Council:

Temperatures and timings for sterilizing with moist heat	
Temperature °C	Timing in minutes
121	15
126	10
134	3

This covers both holding and safety times.

Very large autoclaves are manufactured for commercial and hospital use. For salon use, smaller, simple automatic autoclaves are now manufactured for small-scale sterilization. The required volume of water is placed in the sterilizer. Articles to be sterilized are placed in dishes or on racks within the autoclave. The items must be loaded with care to avoid trapping large bubbles of air, which could interfere with pressure, temperature and timing relationships. Small dishes and vessels should be placed on their side and not inverted. Instruments should be positioned so that steam can contact all surfaces; they should not be placed in bundles. Once the sterilizer is switched on, the cycle is automatically controlled.

Cleaned articles can be loaded at the end of the day and the sterilizer switched on and left to complete its cycle, then unloaded the following morning. Colour-change indicators are available to ensure that sterilizing conditions have been reached.

Disinfectants

Equipment made from materials which are not suitable for sterilization must be disinfected. Also shelves, work surfaces and other surfaces should be regularly wiped over with disinfectant solutions.

A wide variety of products are available, and any information regarding the products should be carefully studied in order to make an informed choice.

Disinfectants must be used in the concentrations and timings recommended; if they are further diluted their effectiveness is reduced. Most disinfectants are more effective at higher temperatures. Other factors which may reduce effectiveness are:

1 The presence of organic matter, such as dead skin, dried blood or vomit; as previously stated, all articles should be cleaned before disinfection.

2 Some disinfectants are inactivated by hard water, while others are inactivated by soaps.

3 Effectiveness is progressively diminished with age. Store only for the recommended time; do not use after expiry date.

Disinfectants, if incorrectly stored, used and diluted, can themselves become infected and be a source of infection.

Examples of disinfectants

■ **Alcohols** such as methanol, ethanol, isopropanol. They form the basis of methylated spirit and surgical spirit. Alcohol is most effective at 70 per cent strength (i.e. seven parts alcohol diluted by three parts water). Bactericidal in action, they kill bacteria but not spores, and their effect against viruses is limited.

Uses: wiping down of all surfaces disinfecting electrodes, ventouse, etc. surgical spirit swabs used on the skin

■ **Aldehydes** such as formaldehyde and glutaraldehyde. Formaldehyde gas is soluble in water and used as formalin. It is highly irritating to tissues and must not be applied to the skin. It is biocidal in action and will destroy bacteria, viruses and fungi and some spores. It is only used in specialized industries.

Glutaraldehyde is an extremely useful disinfectant known as *Cydex*. Germicidal in action, it will kill bacteria, viruses, fungi and most spores if used for a specified length of time. Immersion of over 10 hours would cover everything. It is highly irritating to eyes and skin, and rubber gloves and a surgical mask should be worn when handling this disinfectant.

Uses: Cydex – immersion of instruments and other equipment for disinfection

- **Diguanides** such as chlorhexidine (Hibitane), another good disinfectant. It is less irritating to the skin and eyes than some other disinfectants, but can cause dryness. Effective against bacteria and fungi but less effective against viruses and spores. It is used with detergents in products such as *Hibiscrub*, or with alcohol in products such as *Dispray*.

  Uses: Hibiscrub – hand washing or skin cleansing
  Dispray – cleansing of surfaces

- **Halogens** such as chlorine and iodine. Chlorine is a very effective and cheap disinfectant. It is irritating to eyes and skin and must be used with care as directed. Wear rubber gloves. It is effective against bacteria and some spores and viruses. It is corrosive and not suitable for use on metal instruments. Commercially available products are *Milton* and *Domestos*.

  Uses: Milton – immersion of non-metal instruments, for example those made of plastic or glass
  Domestos – wiping of surfaces, floors, sinks, sanitary ware, etc.; use as directed
  Preparations containing iodine stain the skin brown. They are mainly used as skin disinfectants, but not in beauty therapy.

- **Phenols** such as carbolic acid. Carbolic acid was a very popular antiseptic in the past. It is found in products such as *Lysol* and *Izal*.

  Uses: Izal – cleansing sanitary ware, drains
  Dettol – used on skin
  Dettinox – used to wipe down surfaces

- **Quaternary ammonium compound** are bacteriostatic preventing the multiplication of micro-organisms. Used mainly with detergents for skin and wound cleansing. Found in products such as *Cetavlon* and *Savlon*.

  Uses: cleansing of skin and wounds

Salon Hygiene

This is the responsibility of all therapists and must be taken very seriously. As well as protecting the client, the therapist must protect herself.

Great care must be taken when handling unsterilized sharps and instruments to avoid cuts and stabs which may result in infection. Great care must also be taken when handling disinfectants. These are strong chemicals capable of destroying micro-organisms, but they can also cause damage to the handler, producing burns, etc. When handling these substances, rubber gloves and a surgical mask should always be worn and care taken not to splash the skin, eyes, nose or mouth. Any drops on these areas must be thoroughly rinsed off immediately with cold water.

The following are guidelines which should be followed for establishing high standards of practice and hygiene in the salon.

1 Therapists should wash their hands before and after treatment using a product such as Hibiscrub. Dry with a disposable towel or hot air dryer.

2 The client's skin should be cleaned before treatment using surgical spirit or Savlon wipes. Any cuts must be covered with waterproof plasters.

3 Disposable instruments and equipment should be used whenever possible.

4 Any instrument which pierces the skin should be disposed of and placed in a sharps' box. If this is not practical, then the instrument must be sterilized.

5 All metal instruments should be washed and sterilized, if suitable, using one of the following methods:
(a) Dry heat bead sterilization – this is useful for needles, forceps and other small instruments. However, it is important to remember that any part of the instrument which is not immersed remains unsterilized.
(b) By autoclave (moist heat under pressure) – this is the best method for all articles made of suitable materials.
Metal instruments not suitable for the autoclave must be disinfected in a product which does not cause rusting.

6 All articles that are unsuitable for sterilization must be washed and disinfected. Immerse for the directed time in products such as Cydex, Milton or Barbicide.

7 Articles made from other materials should be cleaned as follows:
(a) **Glass and perspex** Check with manufacturers if the items are suitable for autoclaving as the heat may cause deterioration.
(b) **Vacuum suction (VS) cups** Wash thoroughly with water and detergent using a small brush to reach inaccessible parts, rinse, dry, then immerse for the stated time in Milton, Cydex or Barbicide.
(c) **High frequency electrodes** Keep the metal connecting end dry. Carefully wipe the electrode face with water and detergent, rinse, dry, then wipe over with surgical spirit, wash again and dry.
(d) **Rubber pads** Keep the connecting end dry. Wash carefully with water and detergent, use a soft brush to remove any dirt, rinse and dry. Circles of wet lint or viscose placed between the skin and the electrode will prevent contamination and can be disposed of after treatment or thoroughly washed. Disinfectants can cause deterioration of the rubber and should not be used unless recommended by the manufacturer.
(e) **Viscose or foam pads** Soak and rinse in cold water to remove any chemicals then wash in hot water and detergent, rinse and dry.

8 Working surfaces should be wiped down frequently during the day using 70 per cent alcohol or products such as Dispray. At the end of each day, wash down with water and detergent

and wipe over with 10 per cent Domestos. Chairs, stools, couches and trolleys should also be cleaned in this way at the end of the day.

9   A plentiful supply of good quality towels should be available for covering the couch and for client use. These should be boil washed after each client. Disposable paper sheets should be used to protect the couch cover.

10   Commodities should be chosen with care as creams and lotions, etc., in tubes or narrow-necked bottles have a smaller surface to be contaminated than wide-necked jars.

11   Always use a new clean spatula to remove creams or lotions; do not return any contaminated article back to the product. This is a particular problem when using or applying make-up. Eye shadow, liner, lipstick, powder, etc., should be scraped or removed from the container and placed on a palette. Disposable sponges and cotton wool buds should then be used for applying make-up from the palette. Clients can be encouraged to have their own set of make-up, brushes, etc.

12   A first aid box should be positioned in an obvious, easily accessible place.

13   The stock cupboard should be clean, neat and tidy. Commodities should be clearly labelled showing the use-by date, which should not be exceeded.

14   Bins with plastic liners should be easily reached. All waste should be immediately disposed of; wet waste should first be wrapped in paper. The waste bins should be emptied and disinfected every night and clean liners inserted.

A special sharps' box should be available for disposal of needles, razors, etc., which could penetrate the skin. Special arrangements for the collection and subsequent disposal of these boxes can be organized by contacting the local environmental health officer.

15   Toilet facilities should be easily accessible. These should be well ventilated and disinfected at least once a day. Sanitary ware and floors can be cleaned using Domestos solution.

16   Blood spills must be dealt with immediately. Wear rubber gloves. Pour on neat chlorine (e.g. Domestos), leave for 10 minutes, then wipe off with a disposable cloth. Wash with water and detergent and wipe over with more Domestos.

Personal Hygiene

1   A daily bath or shower will maintain cleanliness of the skin and remove stale sweat, dirt and grease.

2   The use of an antiperspirant after bathing will prevent excessive sweating and the odour of stale sweat.

3   Underwear and tights should be changed daily and washed thoroughly in soapy water, as they absorb body odours.

4   White short-sleeved overalls should be crisp and well laundered. A clean

overall should be worn every other day. Therapists should not wear the uniform out of doors. Outdoor clothing should be changed in a cloakroom to prevent micro-organisms being brought into the salon.

5 Hair must be clean and worn short or tied off the face.

6 The teeth must be cleaned regularly – twice a day; a mouthwash can be used after eating. Smoking or spicy foods should be avoided. Regular dental checks are necessary to prevent the build up of plaque.

7 Hands should receive particular care. They should be washed frequently before and after treatments, after handling any contaminated equipment or using the toilet. A bactericidal soap should be used. A good hand cream should be applied nightly to keep the skin soft and in good condition. Always wear rubber gloves when dealing with blood spills or disinfectants.

8 Nails should be kept short, well manicured and spotlessly clean; organisms can be harboured under the nail. Any nail enamel should be subtle and immaculate – well buffed nails look more natural and any dirt under the nail plate can be quickly seen and removed.

9 Feet should be well cared for. They should be washed and dried thoroughly at least once a day. Talc or foot powder should be used. Nails must be cut regularly, straight across. Well-fitting flat shoes without holes and peeptoes will protect the feet and avoid pressure points.

10 Therapists with colds or any throat infections should not treat clients if possible, but the wearing of a surgical mask will greatly reduce the likelihood of cross infection. Any cuts or infections of the hands or nails should be treated and covered with finger stalls; large areas of infection mean that the therapist should not be working.

11 Food and drink should not be consumed nor stored in the salon working area. Contamination could be transferred to the food and then to the mouth.

Setting up a Salon

The establishment of a hygienic, healthy environment is of prime importance to anyone setting up a salon. Consideration should be given to the following:

1 Rooms should be light, warm and well ventilated.

2 The walls should be covered with a material which can be frequently cleaned and washed down.

3 The floors should be hard, washable surfaces, such as vinyl.

4 Curtains or hangings should be of fabrics that are easy to wash and care for.

5 Couches, chairs, stools, etc., should be covered with smooth, washable materials, such as vinyl or plastic, and kept in good repair.

6 Trolleys, shelves and worktops should be hard, smooth surfaces, free of cracks and easy to clean. They should be kept neat and tidy and uncluttered.

7 There must be handbasins or sinks with a hot water supply so that therapists can wash their hands between treating clients. Hot air dryers or disposable towels should be available for drying.

   A shower should be available for clients to use if required before treatment. All these washing facilities must be kept scrupulously clean.

8 An autoclave should be available for sterilizing instruments.

9 An easily accessible stock cupboard should store clearly labelled commodites.

10 A first aid box must be placed in an obvious, easily accessible position.

11 A bin with a plastic liner should be available in each working area.

12 A plentiful supply of towels should be available. They should be of good quality as they need to be boil washed after each client.

13 A sharps' box must be available and arrangements made for its collection.

14 Good quality products should be used. Those in tubes or ampules are less likely to become contaminated than those in wide-necked jars.

15 Toilet facilities should be easily accessible and kept scrupulously clean.

16 A small cloakroom or large cupboard should be available for hanging outdoor clothes.

SUMMARY

- If micro-organisms invade the body in sufficient numbers to overcome the immune system, they will cause disease.
- Micro-organisms which infect the body are bacteria, viruses, fungi or yeasts and protozoa.

Immunity

- Natural immunity is acquired by previous contact with a disease (the antibodies remain in the body) or acquired via the placenta or milk from the mother.

summary continues overleaf

summary continued from previous page

- Artificial immunity is acquired from vaccines introduced into the body, which stimulate the immune system to produce antibodies, or may be acquired by the transfer of antibodies from a person who has recovered from the disease.
- Bacteria: single cell organisms, non-pathogenic or pathogenic – cocci, bacilli, spirochetes; diseases: boils, impetigo, sore throat, meningitis, pneumonia, typhoid fever, syphilis, cholera.
- Viruses: multiply and destroy the host cells; diseases: colds, influenza, poliomyelitis, mumps, chickenpox, herpes simplex and zoster, warts, hepatitis, HIV.
- Hepatitis and HIV are found in semen, saliva and blood.
- Ways of transmitting a virus: through blood transfusion, drug users sharing needles, the transfer of blood from an infected person into a cut or puncture of the skin, infected women can pass it to the foetus.
- Fungi: yeasts and moulds; diseases: tinea of various parts of body, thrush, fungal infections of organs such as heart and lungs.
- Protozoa: single-celled animals; diseases: sleeping sickness, malaria, amoebic dysentery.
- Parasites live in or on another living organism:
    1 Ectoparasites live outside host (e.g. lice and fleas).
    2 Endoparasites live inside host (e.g. worms and flukes).
- Sterilization is the total destruction of microbes and spores.
- Methods of sterilization in a beauty salon:
    1 Bead sterilizer – small articles only.
    2 Autoclave.
- Disinfecting: the use of a chemical agent which destroys microbes but not spores.
- Disinfectants for use in a salon:
    70 per cent alcohol: methylated spirit and surgical spirit
    isopropyl alcohol
    glutaraldehyde: Cydex
    chlorine: Milton, Domestos
    phenols: Dettol, Dettinox, Izal, Lysol
    ammonium compounds: Cetavlon, Savlon
    diquamides: Hibitane, Hibiscrub, Dispray
- Suggested uses:
    for soaking and immersion of implements: Cydex, Milton and Barbicide
    wiping VS cups and electrodes: surgical spirit, isopropyl, alcohol, Savlon wipes
    cleaning surfaces: Dettinox, Dispray, Domestos
    cleaning skin: surgical spirit, Savlon
    washing hands: Hibiscrub and other bactericidal soaps
    toilets and sanitary ware: Dettol, Izal, Domestos.

QUESTIONS

1   Define the terms 'infection' and 'infestation'.

2   Explain the differences between bacteria and viruses.

3   Give three diseases caused by each of the following:
    (a) bacteria
    (b) viruses
    (c) fungi
    (d) protozoa.

4   Explain the term 'natural immunity'.

5   Give two methods of producing artificial immunity.

6   List the ways in which microbes may enter the body.

7   Explain how microbes may be transmitted.

8   List the forms of the hepatitis virus.

9   Explain how the hepatitis B virus and HIV may be transmitted.

10   Define the terms 'ectoparasite' and 'endoparasite' and give three examples of each.

11   Define the following:
    (a) sterilization
    (b) sanitation
    (c) disinfectant
    (d) antiseptic
    (e) bactericide
    (f) biocide.

12   Identify which of the following are methods of sterilization:
    (a) immersion in Milton
    (b) glass bead boxes
    (c) ultraviolet cabinets
    (d) immersion in Cidex
    (e) autoclaving.

13   Explain how you would deal with the following equipment after use:
    (a) epilation needles
    (b) cuticle knives
    (c) vacuum suction cups
    (d) forceps.

14   List ten factors to be considered for maintaining high standards of salon hygiene.

Ethics, Consultation and Care of the Client

3 Ethics, Planning, Preparation and Client Consultation

OBJECTIVES

After you have studied this chapter you will be able to:

1 Define the term 'Ethics'

2 Discuss the standard of behaviour expected of a professional beauty therapist

3 Explain the importance of client consultation

4 List the essential information which must be recorded on the client consultation

5 Conduct a client consultation

6 Discuss the importance of accurately recording information in accordance with the requirements of the 'Data Protection Act'

7 Explain the importance of, and the procedures involved in, observation and analysis of the client's condition

8 Discuss the importance of accurately identifying the client's condition and problem areas

9 Explain why the evaluation of a treatment is important

10 Prepare the working area, trolley and client for treatment.

Ethics

Ethics refers to the standards and conduct of behaviour of an individual or professional group. Therapists must undergo a course of reputable training to enable them to acquire the understanding and skills necessary to carry out safe and effective treatment. In addition, they must consider their standard of behaviour in relation to colleagues, clients and the general public. In the learning situation the standards and code of behaviour must closely reflect the high standards required in the commercial environment. Training institutions must offer the best facilities and quality tuition, while the students must be diligent and receptive to learning.

Constantly practise the highest ethical standards: this will gain the confidence of clients and establish an excellent reputation which is the basis for success. Prepare yourself before you approach the client and consider the following code of conduct:

1   Look professional – be spotlessly clean, neat and tidy. Maintain the highest standards of personal hygiene and appearance.

2   Be punctual, reliable and keep appointments, do not cancel at the last minute. Always be on time for work and keep to your schedule.

3   Speak clearly, correctly and effectively, adapt the way you communicate to suit the client. Deal politely with everyone, do not use improper language. Consider the manner in which you answer or speak on the telephone. Be competent, helpful and pleasant.

4   Develop a calm, confident and competent attitude. You must feel secure and relaxed in order to transmit this to the client. Clients need to feel that they are in capable hands.

5   Be flexible in your approach to individual clients. You will encounter difficult clients, be courteous at all times even if you feel tired or unwell. Learn to handle tricky situations with tact and diplomacy.

6   Build a good relationship with all the clients. Ask appropriate questions and listen carefully to the answers. Give the client every opportunity to discuss her needs and expectations.

7   Be discreet and refrain from gossip. Remember that clients often confide personal problems during consultation. These facts and all personal details must be treated with the utmost confidentiality. Do not repeat information or gossip to colleagues or others.

8   Be loyal to your employer and colleagues; create a friendly working relationship with everyone.

9   Be honest and reliable, do not make false claims for any treatment but explain the benefits fairly. Be honest when advertising, this will gain you the trust of others and establish a high reputation.

10   Know and abide by legal requirements and local authority by-laws, rules and regulations for conducting your business.

11   Keep up to date with new theories, techniques and treatments. Attend courses on a regular basis and keep in touch with other professionals in your field.

12 Always practise the highest standards of salon hygiene.

13 Ensure that you have sufficient
knowledge, skills and expertise to
advise, select and carry out effective
treatments suited to the needs of
the client.

14 Organize yourself and your business
to ensure a smooth running, efficient service for the benefit of all
concerned.

Planning the Working Day

The efficiency and smooth running of
any organization will depend on good
planning. The therapist must work out
an overall plan for the working day
which will depend on the type and number of appointments booked and she
must plan for each individual treatment.
Working methodically and developing
a good routine while allowing a degree
of flexibility will contribute to the
efficiency of the salon and enhance its
reputation.

■ Arrive early for work, allowing plenty
of preparation time before the first
appointment.

■ Change from outdoor clothes into
your uniform in the changing room.
Check your appearance.

■ Prepare the working area.

■ Check the machines for cleanliness
and safety.

■ Prepare the couch using clean linen,
then cover.

■ Check and prepare other treatment
areas and facilities such as the
UVL (ultraviolet light) cubicle or
exercise area.

■ Check the cloakroom, toilets and
laundry cupboard, etc. Ensure
that everything meets the requirements of the health and safety
legislation.

■ Organize the reception area making
sure that everything is in pristine
order.

■ Check the appointments book and
prepare record cards.

■ Read the notes on the card or
computer for the regular clients
or prepare a new card for new
clients.

■ Behave in a responsible manner at
all times; be friendly and supportive
to other staff and offer help as
required.

Getting to Know the Client

1   When you take on a new client it is important that you get to know each other and establish a good rapport and mutual trust. Meet the client in a friendly, welcoming manner, smile and introduce yourself, use her surname until you get to know her well.

2   Take the initiative, put her at her ease and make her feel comfortable. Be flexible and adaptable in your approach, try and assess the type of person you are dealing with.

3   Find out as much as you can about the client; discuss her needs and what she expects from the treatments.

4   Take her to the treatment area and take time to explain the salon routines. Speak clearly and listen to her responses, make sure that you understand her and that she understands you, be sensitive and supportive to her needs.

5   Watch and be aware of her body language. Her posture, gestures, expressions can tell you a lot about the client. Is she strident, upright, positive, indicating confidence or is she quiet, timid, head hanging, fidgeting, indicating shyness or lack of confidence? Is she familiar with salons and treatments or is this her first experience? Be prepared to adapt your attitude and approach accordingly.

6   Explain the consultation procedure clearly to a new client. Consider the client's modesty and privacy at all times, ask her to undress and remove her jewellery, putting this in her handbag for safe keeping. Give her a robe or towel to wear as appropriate and make sure that she cannot see or be seen by others.

7   Ensure that the client is sitting comfortably. Sit with her, making sure that you have everything that you require for the consultation.

Client consultation

This involves questioning, observation and examination/analysis to assess the client's condition and identify any

Figure 3.1 A client consultation

contraindications to treatment. The assessment must be thorough and accurate and all the facts should be carefully recorded on the client's treatment card.

This information will enable you to set the objectives/goals (what the client wants to achieve as a result of the treatment) and then plan the most beneficial treatment for the client. Remember that this data is the starting point from which future improvements can be measured.

Different consultation procedures will be carried out for facial treatments than for body treatments and different record cards are required. The observation and analysis details will differ but some information will be common to both:

Initial consultation

The consultation is a very important part of the treatment – sufficient time must be allowed so that it is not rushed. This is the time to gather and exchange information. The initial consultation will be the longest and provide detailed information, which must be accurately recorded on a treatment card. This must be filed in a safe and accessible place and used each time the client attends for treatment. Before subsequent treatments, a brief consultation is usually sufficient to establish the effects and outcomes of the previous treatments and whether any changes are to be made or further action is to be taken.

For the consultation the client should be seated comfortably, with the therapist positioned alongside or opposite. The environment should feel warm, well ventilated and private.

Detailed consultation is important for the following reasons:

- To introduce yourself and get to know the client.

- To establish a rapport and put the client at ease.

- To develop mutual trust and gain the client's confidence.

- To gain information on the client's past and present state of mental and physical health.

- To identify any contraindications.

- To gain insight into the client's lifestyle, work environment, leisure activities, etc.

- To identify the client's needs and expectations of the treatment.

- To establish the most appropriate form of treatment and to discuss and agree this with the client.

- To explain the treatment fully to the client, including the procedure, expected effects, timing and frequency.

- To agree a treatment plan, the timing and cost so that the client fully understands the financial commitment, and to obtain a signed consent form.

- To answer queries and questions related to the treatment and to allay doubts and fears.

The information gathered will provide a baseline from which the appropriate treatment is planned, from which the effectiveness of the treatment can be judged and any necessary changes or adjustments made.

All the information given must be recorded and treated in confidence.

Essential information

The following personal, medical and environmental factors should be recorded on the consultation card:

Personal details
- status
- name
- address
- date of birth
- home and work telephone numbers
- occupation
- doctor's name, address and telephone number.

These details will enable you to contact the client quickly should you need to cancel or change an appointment or for any other reason. They will also enable you to seek advice from the client's doctor should this be necessary.

Past medical history
- surgical operations
- pregnancies
- serious illnesses.

These details will enable you to establish the client's state of health; the likelihood of any contraindications as a result of past illnesses; whether particular care must be taken over certain areas and whether medical referral is necessary. If the client suffers from a condition that is an absolute contraindication (see page 56) then treatment must not be given.

Present medical history
- medication
- general health
- current treatments
- identification of stress: work, home or other sources.

These details will indicate whether treatment will be helpful to this client and will influence the type of treatment to be given.

Sample questions to establish physical and emotional condition
- Have you been ill recently – when were you last ill?
- Have you visited the doctor recently?
- Are you on any medication? If so, what medication are you taking?
- Have you suffered any serious illness in the past? If so, what was the problem?
- Have you had any operations in the past or are you awaiting one in the near future?
- Do you suffer from headache, migraine, stress, tension, backache, joint pain or any other problem you want to tell me about?
- Do you suffer from high or low blood pressure, diabetes, epilepsy, psoriasis, eczema or any neurological problems/nervous system disorders?
- Do you have any metal plates or pins inserted? Do you have an electrical implant such as a pacemaker?

- Do you recall any close relative who has suffered from a stroke or heart attack?
- Have you any other problems which I have not mentioned?

Sample questions to establish life style
(You have already found out if your client is married, single, divorced, widowed.)

> The following questions are designed to help you lead the client into a general conversation. Introduce the questions as you pleasantly talk to the client.

- Do you have a family to care for?
- How many children do you have, and how old are they?
- Are they very demanding and require a lot of attention or are they fairly independent?
- Do you go to work?
- What is your occupation?
- What is your daily routine? Are you busy and active all day or are you sitting at a desk for long periods?
- Do you do the cooking, cleaning and all the housework?
- Do you ever feel stressed?
- Do you sleep well every night?
- Do you make time just for yourself each day, to unwind and enjoy yourself?
- What are the ways in which you relax?
- Do you take any form of regular exercise? What activity do you enjoy the most?

- Do you walk regularly, at least three times a week for thirty minutes?
- What is your eating pattern?
- Do you eat regularly?
- Have you ever had an eating problem?
- Are you or have you ever been on a diet?
- Do you eat a healthy balanced diet? Do you eat at least five portions of fruit and vegetables every day with moderate carbohydrate and little fat?
- Do you drink plenty of water or diluted fruit juice, at least 2½ to 3 litres a day?
- Do you drink a lot of coffee? How many cups per day?
- Do you drink alcohol on a regular basis? How many units a week do you drink? (One unit is one glass of wine or half a pint of beer; the recommendation is 7–14 units per week for women and 21 for men.)
- Are you a smoker? How many do you smoke a day? Have you ever tried to give up smoking?
- Do you know that smoking has a detrimental effect on your health and skin?
- Have you attended a beauty salon/health studio before?
- What treatments did you have before? Were they beneficial?
- Which treatment did you enjoy the most?
- Which was the most beneficial?
- How much time can you devote each week to treatments or exercise?

These are a few examples of the questions you can ask to establish a client's lifestyle. You will require further specific questions for facial work and others for body work. Having talked to the client

at length and recorded your findings you now proceed to the looking and testing.

Try writing a list of questions you would ask for facial work and another list for body work.

Contraindications and Contra-actions

Understanding contraindications

Electrical treatments are given to improve specific conditions of the face or body. The treatment must be beneficial and help the client to achieve their desired results. Treatments must not be carried out, even if they are requested by the client if there is any risk of harming the client or making any condition worse.

Every therapist has a legal responsibility under the Health, Safety and Welfare legislation to protect herself and her clients from harm. Remember that if clients are harmed in any way they may make a claim against you. You must therefore ensure that you have not been negligent in any way, that you have selected the appropriate treatment and that you have a written record of the consultation, the treatment given and the aftercare advice.

During the consultation you must decide whether the selected treatment is safe and suitable for the client. If the client is suffering from any condition which could be aggravated or made worse by the treatment, it obviously must not be carried out. These conditions are known as 'contraindications' to treatment. Knowledge of the potentially harmful effects of

inappropriate treatment is extremely important and so is the ability to recognize contraindications.

The effects of the treatment may be harmful in certain circumstances. The following explanations will help you to understand why some treatments should not be carried out if certain conditions are present. There are dangers associated with the following.

Cardiovascular problems

An increase in blood flow may be desirable in many conditions, but can be undesirable and even dangerous in others. Heart conditions, high and low blood pressure will mean that certain treatments should not be carried out. All heat treatments should be avoided as they increase the heart rate and lower blood pressure.

Bruising, damaged or broken blood vessels may be further damaged by the treatment resulting in increased bleeding. Bruises must be allowed to heal before treatment.

Varicose veins should be avoided as the tissues around the vein may be fragile and easily damaged. There is a tendency for the stagnating blood to form clots which may be dislodged by the treatment.

Thrombosis or phlebitis Avoid treatment if a client suffers from either or both of these conditions (known as **thrombophlebitis.**

If a vein in the calf becomes inflamed (phlebitis), treatment may increase the inflammation but the greatest danger lies if a clot develops in the vein (thrombosis). If the circulating blood slows down, platelets and fibrin adhere to the vessel wall forming a clot. While the clot is attached to the vessel wall it is called a **thrombus**. If the clot or a portion of it breaks off and becomes dislodged, is called an **embolism**. This will move through the blood stream and may cause a blockage in a smaller vein, cutting off the blood supply to the area beyond the blockage. If this blockage occurs in the lungs or brain it could be fatal.

Dislodging or fragmenting a blood clot is the greatest danger of treatments to the legs as death could result if medical treatment is not administered quickly.

Thrombosis usually develops in the calf or hamstrings. Be alert and suspect this condition if a client complains of deep pain in the calf or back of the thigh. There may be swelling of the area and the muscles may feel tense and hard. Refer to a doctor or hospital immediately.

Infections and cancer cells can be carried from one part to another part of the body in the blood or lymph.

The lymphatic system removes excess fluid from all over the body returning it into the blood stream. Lymph transports the larger particles of waste from the tissues as well as bacteria, viruses or cancerous substances. Because treatments increase the lymphatic flow, the rate at which these toxic substances are carried and spread around the body is increased.

Be particularly aware if the client has a temperature, swollen painful joints or painful swellings in lymph glands: do not treat and seek medical advice.

Skin diseases and wounds

Infections may be transmitted from client to therapist or from therapist to client through touch or may be spread from an infected area to a non-infected area. This is why careful and thorough washing of hands, covering of any skin breakages and sterilizing equipment is so important.

When you touch a client's skin, any bacterial, viral or fungal infection can be spread over the skin to a non-infected area or on to your hands. Any infection on your hands can be transmitted to the client. Electrodes may also spread infections. Friction of the hands or equipment may open healing wounds or abrasions. This will expose the area to infection by micro-organisms.

With open wounds there will be a risk of blood contamination between the client and the therapist. Blood contamination must be avoided as serious life-threatening viruses and diseases such as Hepititis B and HIV (Aids) can be transmitted in this way. (Remember that infection may pass from client to client via the commodities such as pillows, towels, sheets, etc. Infestation by parasites such as lice, flees and itch mites can be passed in the same way.)

Tissue injuries and recent scar tissue

Any injury or damage to the tissues or fractures of bones or recent scar tissue must be allowed to heal completely before treatment is given to the area.

If treatment is given before healing is complete, there is a danger of further damage to the tissues delaying the healing process. There is a risk of breaking down recent scar tissue.

Pins and plates

If treatment is performed over an area where pins and plates have been inserted to stabilize bones and joints, there is a danger that vigorous movement may loosen them or if they protrude there is a danger of damaging the surrounding soft tissues.

Sensitive skin and sunburn

Clients with sensitive skin must not receive stimulating treatments as these will exacerbate the condition. The erythema (reddening) following sunburn must clear completely before treatment can be given.

The products used for treatments may cause an allergic reaction in some clients. This will produce an excessive erythema, the area becoming very red and hot or a rash may appear. Remove the medium immediately and wash in warm water.

Fragile loose skin

There is a danger of overstretching loose skin and of breaking down fragile, thin skin causing open wounds.

Particular care must be taken with diabetics and anyone on steroid treatments as the skin may be fragile and healing may be slow. Superficial treatments with light pressure only must be used.

Lack of skin sensitivity

The hot/cold and sharp/blunt sensitivity test is an important part of any consultation.

The hot/cold test is essential prior to heat treatments as you need to know whether the client can feel the heat.

The sharp/blunt test is essential for all treatments where the client needs to tell you that the current is felt.

Both tests are essential for all galvanic treatments as the client must report any build up of heat (hot spots) and must report if the intensity of the current is too high.

Epilepsy and diabetes

Clients with these conditions require particular care. Although epilepsy is usually well controlled with medication, the client should be observed at all times as there is a risk of seizure which may result in a fall or other injury.

Clients with diabetes may have impaired sensitivity, poor circulation and healing may be slow. Great care must be taken to avoid damage to the skin or any other injury.

Conditions where treatment is contraindicated

Definitions

A **contraindication** is a condition which, if present, means that the treatment should not be carried out.

Some conditions mean that treatment is totally contraindicated and must not be performed to any part of the body. These are known as **absolute contraindications.**

Other conditions prevent treatment over the local area of the condition, but other non-affected areas or limbs may be treated, these are known as **local contraindications.**

Absolute contraindications to electrical treatments

Do not treat a client if any of the following contraindications are present.

- **Cancer**: any client with cancer or a history of cancer must not be treated as there may be a risk of cancer cells being carried to other parts of the body via the circulating blood or the lymphatic system. If you are unsure seek medical advice.

    Be particularly aware if a client complains of intractable pain on rest, unexplained loss of weight, feeling generally tired or unwell.

- **Acute infectious disease and fever**: if the client feels hot, feverish, is perspiring and generally unwell.

- **Nausea**: if the client is feeling sick or has a severe headache .

- **Dysfunction or disorders of the nervous system**: such as multiple sclerosis, strokes, Parkinson's disease, etc., when the conductivity of nerve impulses may be abnormal; where muscles may exhibit increased tone (spasticity) which may be made worse by the treatment; where skin sensation may be impaired. These clients must only be treated if medically directed in a medical clinic.

- **Drink or drugs**: treatment must not be given to anyone under the influence of drink or drugs as such a client may not be in control of their faculties.

- **Inflammatory disease**: when the client is in the active phase of any inflammatory disease such as rheumatoid arthritis or any area which is red, hot and swollen.

- **Pregnancy**: in the late stages of pregnancy or if the client is experiencing any problems with her pregnancy seek medical advice.

- **Haemophilia**: a condition of diminished or absence of blood clotting. Anyone suffering from this condition will bruise and bleed easily, and should not be treated.

- **Phlebitis and thrombosis**: phlebitis is a painful condition where the lining of the vein becomes inflamed and may result in a clot forming on the vein wall, known as thrombosis. Any pressure applied to the vein or increase in the force of the circulation may dislodge the clot. The embolism will then be carried in the blood stream with potentially fatal consequences.

The danger of treating a client with these conditions is explained above. Treatment of the legs is a definite contraindication and it is safer not to treat the body as there will always be a slight risk. Facial treatments may be carried out with care.

Local contraindications for each treatment are listed in the individual chapters. Explanations covering these contraindications are provided in the preceding section.

Contra-actions

These are conditions which may arise during the treatment which would indicate that the treatment must stop. During treatment be alert to any abnormal changes happening to the client which mean that you should not continue with the treatment. These conditions include:

- headache
- nausea
- vomiting
- profuse sweating
- restlessness and irritability
- feeling faint
- abnormal erythema
- the area becoming very hot and red
- stomach or any abdominal pain
- joint pain
- muscle fatigue
- galvanic burns
- bruising.

If any of these conditions arise, remove any products, slowly place the client in the recovery position and allow the client to rest for 10 minutes or so. Stay with the client until she or he feels better. Allow the client to sit up slowly and rest in this position. If there is still cause for concern seek advice from the person responsible for first aid.

Observation and Analysis

Place the client in a suitable position for the examination/analysis to take place and consider her comfort and modesty at all times. Explain each step fully, encourage the client to ask questions and answer her clearly. It is most important that she knows and understands what you are doing and why it is necessary.

For facial work you will carry out a full skin analysis. You will study the skin type, skin condition and colour, you will assess muscle tone and study the contours of the face, you will also look for contraindications.

For body work you will assess through observation and manual examination the body type, the distribution of body fat, any evidence of fluid retention and the degree of muscle tone. You will also carry out a detailed examination of posture and look for contraindications.

When contraindications are identified or when in doubt as to whether treatment should be carried out then you must seek the doctor's consent. Be very tactful when suggesting this, do not name the condition nor alarm the client. Remember that the doctor is the only person qualified to make a diagnosis and to inform the client. You may have recognized a condition but you could be wrong. You need only say, 'I am not sure whether this condition is suitable for this treatment, so would you mind checking with your doctor?' The salon will probably have a standard letter which you can fill in and which simply requires the doctor's signature.

You may also need to carry out a skin sensitivity test, depending on treatment selection.

Skin analysis prior to facial treatment	Body analysis prior to body treatment
Skin type	Body type
Skin condition	Posture
Skin colour	Distribution of soft and hard fat
Blemishes	Areas of cellulite
Facial contours	Testing for muscle tone
Muscle tone	Areas of fluid retention
Contraindications	Skin condition
	Contraindications

Selecting the Treatment

Having completed a detailed analysis and examination you will have identified the problem areas. Discuss your findings tactfully with the client and ask her if she agrees with your assessment. You must then agree the outcomes/goals and select the treatment. It is vitally important that you accurately identify the client's condition and select the most suitable and effective treatment, as the result you achieve will depend on this.

You will require an in-depth knowledge of all the equipment, treatments and products at your disposal so that you can make an informed choice. As a student, remembering all the treatments may be quite difficult while you are just starting. It is therefore a good idea to list on a card the different facial conditions with all available suitable treatments and on the reverse side to list the body conditions with all appropriate treatments. This can be kept in your pocket and referred to if you are uncertain – but do this out of sight of the client!

Once you have decided upon the best treatment possible you must discuss it fully with the client giving reasons why you consider it to be the most suitable and beneficial treatment for her.

You must then discuss the *timing* of each session, the *number* of sessions recommended per week, the *length* of the course and most important of all, the *cost* per session including cost of any recommended products. Most salons offer an incentive for a course of treatment – this may include free products or the offer of two free sessions at the end of the course.

Make sure that the client understands her commitment, encourage her to ask questions and answer her fully. You must agree everything with the client and when she is satisfied make sure that she signs an agreement/consent form.

Carrying out the Treatment

Any treatment must be carried out skilfully and with care. Always practise the highest standards of hygiene and safety. Do your very best for every client, explain each procedure as you go along and check that the client is happy and comfortable throughout. Time the treatment carefully giving each area equal attention, aim to complete the treatment in the allocated time span. Be on the alert for any contra-actions that may arise during treatment such as excessive erythema, allergic reactions, fainting, nosebleeds, breathing difficulties, nausea, vomiting, headache, muscle fatigue, galvanic burns or bruising. Any one of these conditions means that the treatment must stop and appropriate action taken.

Section 4 will give the underpinning information and the details of preparation, procedure and technique for each treatment.

Evaluation of treatment

After each treatment it is important to assess how effective the treatment has been. You must decide whether the treatment has produced the effects that you were expecting, and whether the goals you set at the beginning have been met.

In order to evaluate the treatment you will need to obtain feedback: this means gathering all the information you can which will indicate the effectiveness of the treatment. Knowledge of the results of the treatment will enable you to make changes or modifications next time should you feel that you have not achieved your goal. You will obtain information through touch, that is sensing through your hands whether the tissues feel more toned; You will also obtain information by looking at the area to see what changes have been produced. You will acquire more information through asking the client how she feels and whether the treatment met her needs.

As a result of the information you obtain from this feedback you will decide if changes need to be made and formulate a strategy for the next treatment. You have to make a judgement as to whether your selected treatment has been as effective as you hoped.

Through **palpating** the tissues you will sense whether the tissues feel more relaxed:

- Are the tissues firmer?
- Are the tissues more flexible and smoother?
- Do the tissues feel warm but not too hot?

By **looking** at and **examining** the area you will obtain visual feedback:

- Is there a good even erythema?
- Are there uneven patches of erythema which would suggest uneven pressure?
- Does the skin look brighter, cleaner, more refined ?
- Is the area very red and hot which would indicate over-treating or a mild allergic reaction to the product?
- Are there red sore spots over bony prominences indicating that these were not avoided?

By **questioning** the client you will obtain verbal feedback:

- How did that feel?
- Did you enjoy the treatment?
- Did any part of the treatment feel uncomfortable?
- Did it hurt at any time?
- Was the current/heat comfortable throughout?
- Did you understand my explanation of the treatment and was it as you expected it to be?
- Were you nervous or anxious at any time?
- Did you feel relaxed or go to sleep?
- Was the treatment even and equal on both sides?

- Did you feel that you would have liked me to spend a longer time on any area?
- Was there any area that you would prefer me to leave out next time?
- Do you feel entirely satisfied with the treatment?

Allow the client time to relax and get up slowly. Discuss any changes that you intend making next time and explain the reasons why they are needed and ask if there is anything the client would like to change. Record the results of the feedback and the strategy for following treatments on the record card:

- Always refer to these each time the client attends.
- Give home advice as appropriate.

Advice and After Care

The client must be given advice and guidance on the routine to follow immediately after treatment and in the interval between treatments. The advice given will obviously vary depending on the treatment given.

Examples

- Following certain facial treatments the client should not wear make-up for 24 hours.
- The client should be advised on skin care and a suitable make-up routine to follow between treatments.

- After UVL irradiation, treatments must be avoided until the erythema has subsided.
- After heat treatments the client should shower, rest and replenish fluids.
- Following body treatments the client should be shown suitable exercises to be done at home.
- Dietary advice may be offered when appropriate.
- The client may need to be taught relaxation techniques.
- Advice and instruction on correct breathing techniques may be required.

Relaxation

Relaxation means being free from the tension and anxiety which are normally caused by the stresses of life and which upset the body balance. It is impossible to remove all the stressors in life and a certain amount of stress is desirable as it can produce feelings of thrill and excitement. The ability to relax is extremely important as it combats stress and reduces its harmful effects such as fatigue, lethargy, illness and psychological problems. Clients who lead very busy lives or are coping with worries or dealing with unhappy situations may find it very difficult to relax. Advising them and showing them ways of reducing stress and promoting relaxation can form an important part of treatment. Once they have recognized the difference between the tense state and the relaxed state they can continue to practise at home.

Preparation

The first consideration is to prepare the room or cubicle and create the right conditions to promote the relaxation response, namely:

- A warm, well ventilated area.

- A quiet area, away from distracting noise.

- Low and diffused lighting.

- A spotlessly clean environment.

- Soothing décor in pastel colours.

- A comfortable couch or mattress on the floor.

- Clean linen and towels for every client; these to be boil washed after each use.

- Light blankets for additional warmth.

- Very soft, slow moving music may be played if the client dislikes absolute quiet.

Relaxation techniques

There are many techniques which may be used to encourage the client to relax. They may be combined for maximum effect.

The relaxation response involves the client's response to a quiet soothing environment and total concentration on a particular object while trying to let go of all tension. This is sometimes sufficient to promote the relaxed state and can be practised anywhere.

Visualization or imagery involves visualizing pleasantly soothing situations conducive to relaxation (e.g. lying on a beach; looking at a tranquil scene, etc.).

Progressive relaxation aims to develop an awareness of the difference between feelings of tension and relaxation. Contraction followed by relaxation of all the muscle groups is performed, working around the body. This is a very effective method of promoting relaxation.

Progressive relaxation technique

Select and prepare a suitable area and prepare the client (see page 67).

The client should lie on a mattress and be fully supported. The client may choose to lie on the back, in the recovery position or half-lying if the client has difficulty in lying flat. The client must be well supported using plenty of pillows under the head, knees or as required. Allow the client a short time to settle and let go of tension. During this time encourage the client to breath deeply and let go when breathing out.

The technique is then practised as follows, beginning with the feet and repeating each movement three times.

1 Pull the feet up hard (**dorsiflexion**) and let go.
2 Push the feet down hard (**plantar flexion**) and let go.
3 Push the knees down hard against the floor and let go.
4 Push the leg down hard against the floor and let go.
5 Tighten the buttock muscles hard and let go.
6 Pull the abdominal muscles in hard and let go.
7 Raise the shoulders and let go.
8 Press the shoulders into the floor and let go.
9 Press the arms into the floor and let go.
10 Curl the fingers to make a fist and let go.
11 Press the head into the floor and let go.
12 Screw up and tighten the face and let go.
13 Tighten all the groups together and let go.

The client should breathe out on the 'let go'.

Use your voice to encourage relaxation when teaching these movements. The command 'tighten hard' can be used after each instruction with a firm voice, while 'let go' should be spoken in a lower tone and drawn out to encourage the feeling of letting go. The terms 'relax' or 'release' may be used in place of 'let go'.

The clients should be left to repeat the sequence on their own until they feel free of tension and sleepy. They may be allowed to sleep, time permitting, and woken up slowly. This sequence can be practised at home in a quiet place, it is particularly effective after taking a warm bath.

Breathing exercises

Breathing exercises are given to maintain and improve the expansion of the chest. This increases the amount of oxygen taken into the lungs and increases the amount of carbon dioxide out of the lungs. Breathing in is known as **inspiration**, and breathing out is known as **expiration**. The muscles of respiration are the external intercostal muscles, the internal intercostal muscles which lie between the ribs and the diaphragm which lies horizontally separating the thoracic cavity from the abdominal cavity. The contraction of these muscles will increase the capacity of the thorax from side to side, from front to back and longitudinally from top to bottom.

Effects of breathing exercises

- Improve the mobility of the thorax.
- Increase the intake of the oxygen which will improve metabolism.
- Increase the output of carbon dioxide, thus eliminating this waste product more quickly.
- Improve the condition of the lungs.
- Loosening lung secretions.

- The changing pressure created in the thorax aids the flow of blood in the veins and the flow of lymph in the lymphatic vessels.

- The increased mobility of the thorax improves posture.

Technique

Position: sitting on a chair or lying. Remove any tight restricting clothing.

Deep breathing concentrates on three areas of expansion, namely: apical, costal and diaphragmatic.

Apical breathing Place the hands on the upper chest below the clavicle, breathe in deeply through the nose and expand the chest under the hands. The chest will move up and forward as you breathe in; then breathe out through the mouth and the chest will move back as you breathe out. Try not to allow movement in the other parts of the chest. Repeat three times.

Costal breathing Place the hands on the side of the ribs, above the waist. Breathe in deeply through the nose and feel the ribs moving out sideways; breathe out through the mouth and the ribs will move back as you breathe out. Repeat three times.

Diaphragmatic breathing Place the hands in front, above the waist. Breath in deeply through the nose and feel the lower chest and abdomen moving forward as you breathe in; breathe out through the mouth and pull the abdomen back in as you breathe out. Repeat three times.

Then breathe deeply using all areas of the chest as follows: breathe in deeply through the nose, hold to a count of five and breathe out for as long as possible through the mouth. Repeat three times.

Practise yourself before teaching clients to ensure that you fully understand the movements. Deep breathing can make one feel dizzy and faint because the amount of oxygen and carbon dioxide in the body is changing and the balance between these chemicals is disturbed. If this occurs then it is important to rest for a few minutes until the feeling passes and the balance is restored. This must be explained to clients before they are encouraged to practise at home.

Preparation for Treatment

Preparation of working area

- Ensure that the working area affords the client total privacy to change and receive treatment without being overlooked by others. The area may be a curtained section in a large salon, an individual walled cubicle or a small treatment room.

The therapist should ensure there is enough space to walk around the bed and work from all sides and that there is room for a trolley with commodities, the equipment and a stool.

- The environment should be warm, well-ventilated and draught free.

- It should be quiet, peaceful and free from distracting noise. Soft relaxing music may be played, but check with the client – some clients prefer quiet.
- The lighting should be soft and diffuse, not directed from above and shining into the client's face.
- The colour scheme should be pale but warming, using pastel rather than harsh bold colours.
- The area must be spotlessly clean and tidy.
- Items required during the treatment must be neatly arranged on the trolley shelf and protected with clean paper tissue or a small sheet.
- A plentiful supply of clean laundered towels and linen should be to hand.
- Extra pillows, small support pillows or rolled towels should also be to hand.
- Shower and toilet facilities for the client should be accessible and regularly cleaned. A hand basin or sink should be available for washing the therapist's hands. Disposable towels or hot air dryers should be used to dry the hands. These must all be scrupulously clean.
- A lined bin should be to hand for disposal of waste.

Preparation of treatment couch

Prepare the couch before the client arrives:

- Cover the entire surface with a towelling or cotton sheet – the fitted types are best as they stay neat and tidy.

- Next cover this with a large bath towel or cotton sheet. This must be removed and boil washed after each client and a clean one reapplied. Many salons and colleges use disposable paper sheets (bed roll) to save on the laundry – these are quite acceptable, but they can tear and crumple during the treatment.
- Use one or two pillows for the head. Cover these with pillow slips and then a towel.
- Fold two large towels and place them at the foot of the bed. These will be used to cover the client as required.
- Place extra pillows, large and small, on the trolley for use if extra support is required during the treatment.
- Make sure that the couch is at the correct height. A couch that is too high will result in a strain on the arms, neck and shoulders, a couch which is too low will result in back strain.

You must make sure that you protect yourself from strains or any damage as a result of poor posture or poor lifting techniques.

Preparation of trolley or table

- Select a trolley or table with a hard, smooth surface, free of cracks and easy to clean. Ensure that it is robust and sturdy so that it cannot be pushed over. Wheels are an advantage as the trolley may be pulled or pushed into a convenient position.
- Place the trolley near the treatment couch so that all items will be to hand

when required. Ensure that the trolley is large enough to safely support the equipment.

- The trolley and electrical equipment should be placed on your dominant side, on the right if you are right-handed and on the left if you are left-handed. This avoids reaching over the client to adjust the controls.

- Wipe the shelves with disinfectant of the correct dilution.

- Cover the shelves with paper sheets – fold under all edges for neatness.

- Position the machine on the trolley unless it is free standing and arrange cleaned bottles and bowls neatly. Always place commodities in the same order to ensure that they are easy to identify and reach when needed. Plastic baskets may be used to hold the bottles neatly. Clean these with disinfectant before loading.

- A bowl for waste, lined with clean disposable tissue, should be placed on a lower shelf, or a bin with a disposable liner may be placed under the trolley. This is to avoid the risk of contamination of the commodities.

- Cover the shelf and commodities with a clean paper sheet when not in use. This will protect items from dust and dirt.

- At the end of each day strip the trolley down; wipe the shelves with disinfectant; clean all the bottles and bowls, then either store the commodities in a cupboard ready for use the following day or re-lay the trolley and cover.

Preparation of the therapist

Before carrying out a treatment therapists must prepare themselves physically, paying due consideration to high standards of professionalism and hygiene. Cleanliness is essential to protect both the client and the therapist from cross infection. They must also prepare psychologically and give due thought to the type of treatment required.

Personal hygiene

- A daily bath or shower should be taken to maintain cleanliness of the skin, hair and nails and to remove stale sweat odours.

- An antiperspirant should be used to prevent excessive sweating and the odour of stale sweat.

- Hair should be clean and neat; it should be kept short or tied back from the face. Hair must never fall forward around the therapist's face and shoulders or touch the client.

- Nails must be well manicured and kept short; nails should not protrude above the fleshy part of the finger tip as long nails may harbour dirt and micro-organisms. Nail enamel should not be worn as some clients may be sensitive to the product and an allergic reaction may result. Enamel would also hide dirt under the nails.

- Hands must be well cared for; they must be smooth and warm. Therapists should protect the hands with rubber gloves when doing chores. A good-quality hand lotion should be used night and morning. Gloves should be worn in cold weather.

Therapists should not carry out treatments with cuts or abrasions on the hands. Small areas may be covered with a waterproof plaster and fingerstall.

- Jewellery should be removed or kept to a minimum of wedding ring and small ear studs. Rings, bracelets and watches can harbour micro-organisms or can injure the client if dragged on the skin. Long earrings and necklaces may jangle, producing a noise that is disturbing to the client.

- Underwear and tights should be changed daily and washed in hot soapy water.

- White, short-sleeved overalls should be crisp, well laundered and changed frequently (e.g. every other day). The style should allow free unrestricted movement of the arms during treatments.

- Feet should be well cared for and washed and dried thoroughly once a day, using foot powder if necessary. A clean pair of tights should be worn each day: support tights will help prevent tired legs and varicose veins. Well-fitting low-heeled or flat shoes without holes or peeptoes will protect the feet and avoid pressure points.

- Working uniform should not be worn out of the salon. Outdoor clothing worn to work should be changed in a cloakroom to prevent micro-organisms being brought into the salon.

- Therapists suffering from colds and infections should not treat clients if possible, but the wearing of a surgical mask will greatly reduce the risk of cross infection.

- Therapists must wash their hands frequently, particularly before touching a client, after carrying out cleansing procedures and at the end of every treatment.

- Teeth must be cleaned regularly and breath must be kept free from odours.

Preparation of the client

- Speak to the client in a polite and friendly manner, introduce yourself and make the client feel at ease.

- Maintain client privacy at all times.

- Show the client the treatment area and shower room, explain how to operate the shower.

- Ask the client to undress and provide a robe or towel to wear.

- Ask the client to remove all jewellery and place it in her bag for safe keeping.

- Bring the client back to the treatment area and make her comfortable.

- Carry out the client consultation and assessment.

- Discuss your recommended treatment with the client. Explain the benefits and procedure. Allow time for the client to discuss any problems or ask questions and answer these fully.

- Always help the client on and off the bed, this will ensure that she cannot fall and injure herself.

- Position the client correctly on the couch, make sure that she is well supported and relaxed.

■ Cover the client and make sure that she is warm and comfortable.

Positioning the client

Finally, the following checklist concerns the techniques for positioning the client in the salon during treatment.

Positioning the client on the bed or couch

■ The bed should be prepared in advance.
■ Cover with a clean towel or fitted cover.
■ Cover pillows with a clean towel.
■ Cover the bed and pillows with disposable paper sheet (bed roll).
■ Two towels should be provided to cover the client. Blankets may be used over the towel if the client feels cold, however they are difficult to launder and should not come in contact with the client.
■ A supply of extra pillows and towels should be available for extra support when necessary.

The position of the client will depend on the treatment. Clients may be placed:

■ **Prone** lying (face down).
■ **Supine** lying (face up) or half-lying (back raised at an angle).
■ **Recovery position** on the side, lying with under arm and leg behind and upper arm and leg bent to support the body.

In the prone position it is more comfortable for the client if the feet project over the edge of the bed. This prevents stretching of the ligaments at the front of the ankle. The head may be turned to one side. A pillow under the abdomen may be more comfortable and will round out a hollow back.

In the supine or half-lying position, a pillow to support the head will improve comfort. A pillow under the knees and thighs will also improve comfort and aid relaxation.

In the recovery position a pillow under the head and a pillow supporting the upper leg improve comfort.

Figure 3.2 Prone lying

Figure 3.3 Supine lying

Figure 3.4 Recovery position

Recording Details

1 Develop the habit of accurately and neatly recording all the details as you progress through each stage. Do not leave it until the end as important information may be forgotten.

   All the information you have gathered and stored is confidential. It is important that this confidentiality is maintained in accordance with the Data Protection Act (1998).

2 If you exceed the time allocated, analyse why and make adjustments next time.

3 You will be required to produce examples of these records of treatment in your evidence portfolio. The information can be supported by notes, tapes or video recordings of the consultation. These can show how you approached different types of clients, how you discussed various issues with them or how you dealt with problems or tricky situations. The evidence can illustrate how you obtained help from superiors or colleagues when necessary and how skilfully you carried out the treatment, observing hygiene and safety standards. You could also include photographs of before and after treatments.

You can follow but adapt this planning format for all the treatments covered in this book.

Evaluation of Own Performance

To judge how you have performed, ask yourself the following questions:

- Did I check and ensure that my uniform, hair, nails, footwear and appearance were immaculate?

- Did I make sure that everything was in place prior to the client's arrival? That is, the room (to ensure a suitable, quiet environment), the couch (clean linen, towels and pillows), the trolley (neatly laid out with all commodities to hand).

- Did I abide by the salon's health, safety and hygiene policies?

- Did I adopt a friendly, relaxed, professional, competent manner?

- Did I respect the client's privacy and dignity?

- Did I observe the client's body language?

- Did I adapt my approach to suit the type of client?

- Did I make the client feel at ease?

- Did I communicate well with the client, was I polite, sensitive and supportive?

- Did I carry out a detailed client consultation and record the information on a treatment card and get it signed by the client?

■ Did I note all contraindications and take the required action?

■ Did I allow the client the opportunity and time to express her needs and expectations?

■ Did I listen closely to what she was saying?

■ Did I select the most suitable treatment and set long-term goals?

■ Did I explain everything clearly to the client and did she understand my explanation?

■ Did I agree the treatment plan, cost and timing with the client and obtain her written consent?

■ Did I maintain eye contact with the client?

■ Was I aware of my own body language?

■ Did I make the client feel secure, comfortable and cared for?

■ Did I select the best possible treatment to suit the client?

■ Did I select the most suitable product and make sure I did not waste any?

■ Did I wash my hands before touching the client and after treatment ?

■ Did I adopt the correct posture and position to avoid strain, injury and fatigue?

■ Did I check the safety of the electrical equipment: plugs, cable, leads, terminals?

■ Did I check the current and ensure that the intensity was at zero?

■ Did I check the well-being of the client during the treatment?

■ Did I evaluate the treatment outcomes?

■ Did I offer home advice?

■ Did I keep within the time constraints for a viable cost-effective treatment?

■ Did I dispose of all waste into a lined bin with a lid?

■ Did I clean the treatment area and leave it tidy?

This list will also help you to prepare for assessment as these are pointers to successful performance.

QUESTIONS

1   List any six practices which illustrate and maintain high ethical standards.
2   Give ten reasons why a detailed consultation is important.
3   Briefly explain the procedures you would follow when you arrive at work in preparation for the working day.
4   Give the information required on a client treatment record card.
5   Briefly explain the features you would examine during a body analysis prior to any body treatment.
6   Briefly explain the features you would examine during a skin analysis prior to any facial treatment.
7   List the factors which must be explained and discussed with the client after you have selected the treatment and prior to commencement of the treatment.
8   Discuss how verbal and visual feedback aids the evaluation of the treatment.
9   Give five factors which encourage relaxation which you would consider when you are preparing the working area.
10 Briefly discuss the preparation of the client prior to treatment.

Underpinning Science

4 Basic Science

OBJECTIVES

After you have studied this chapter you will be able to:

1 List the three states of matter.

2 Differentiate between an element and a compound.

3 Describe the structure of an atom.

4 Discuss the formation of **ions** and explain the terms **cation** and **anion**.

5 Describe the flow of electrons through a conductor.

6 Differentiate between conductors and non-conductors (insulators).

7 Define and draw a graphical illustration of the following:

(a) direct current

(b) alternating current

(c) high frequency current.

8 Explain the following electrical units:

(a) amps

(b) ohms

(c) volts

(d) watts.

9 Define Ohm's law and use it for calculations.

10 Calculate the cost of electricity by reading the meter for number of units used.

11 Distinguish between closed circuit, open circuit and short circuit.

12 Explain how the following devices modify current:

(a) transformer

(b) rectifier

(c) capacitor.

13 Discuss the replacement of 'blown' fuses.

14 Explain the procedure to be followed when rewiring a plug.

Figure 4.1   Portable high frequency and galvanic unit

This chapter deals with basic science which is relevant to the beauty therapist. It is suggested that all students study this chapter before embarking on electrical treatments as it will provide a background knowledge of atoms, ions, basic electricity, conductors, electrical units, Ohm's law, devices for modifying current, types of current and circuits. Where relevant, further scientific theory is to be found at the beginning of each chapter.

States of Matter

Everything around us is composed of matter and all matter is made up of small particles called atoms. Matter can exist in any one of three states depending on temperature and pressure. The three states of matter are:

1 solid

2 liquid

3 gas.

> Matter can exist as a solid, liquid or gas depending on temperature and pressure.

In the solid state, the particles are tightly packed and regularly arranged and move or vibrate only slightly; solids are very dense. In the liquid state, the particles are more widely spaced and move more freely; liquids are usually less dense than solids (ice being one exception). In the gaseous state, the particles are very widely spaced and move at high speed; gases have a lower density than liquids and solids.

If a solid is heated beyond its melting point it will form a liquid, and if a liquid is heated beyond its boiling point it will form a gas. The converse is also true: if a gas is cooled it will condense to form a liquid, and if a liquid is cooled it will form a solid.

Solid

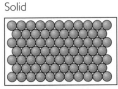

Particles have a regular
pattern, are close
together, they move
slightly and have high
density

Liquid

Particles are more
widely spaced, move
more freely and have a
medium density

Gas

Particles are widely
spaced, move randomly
at high speed and have
a low density

Figure 4.2   Particles in a solid, liquid and gas

Elements

Matter is made up of chemical **elements** and their various compounds. An element is a substance in its simplest form which cannot be further broken down by chemical reaction.

There are 109 known elements, and about 90 of these occur naturally. At room temperature and pressure, most elements are solid and metallic (e.g. copper, iron); some are liquid (e.g. mercury, bromine) and some are gases (e.g. hydrogen, oxygen).

Common elements	
Metal	Non-metal
Copper	Oxygen
Iron	Nitrogen
Zinc	Carbon
Sodium	Chlorine
Potassium	Sulphur
Calcium	

Elements can combine to form compounds.

Compounds

Elements can combine and react together to form **compounds**. The properties of the compound will be different from the properties of the individual elements from which it is made, for example, the elements hydrogen and oxygen react to form the compound water.

Each element can be represented in shorthand by a symbol usually made up of one or two letters, for example:

Hydrogen: H   Calcium: Ca
Oxygen: O   Chlorine: Cl
Potassium: K   Sodium: Na

When two elements join together to form a compound, the symbols are combined, for example:

Sodium + chlorine $\rightarrow$ Sodium chloride

$Na^+ + Cl^-$ $\rightarrow$ NaCl

Atomic Structure

Elements are made up of atoms. An atom is the smallest part of an element that retains its distinct chemical properties and that can take part in a chemical reaction. Atoms are made up of even smaller particles, the main ones being protons, electrons and neutrons.

> An atom is the smallest part of an element that can take part in a chemical reaction.

Two of these subatomic particles carry an electrical charge: protons have a positive charge; electrons have a negative charge; neutrons have no charge, that is they are neutral.

All the atoms of one element are identical and contain the same numbers of these particles (e.g. all atoms of helium have two electrons, two protons and two neutrons). Atoms of different elements have different numbers of particles. The arrangement of these particles in an atom follows a definite pattern.

In each atom the protons and neutrons are tightly packed together in the nucleus of the atom. The electrons orbit around the nucleus in distinct energy levels or electron shells. Each orbit or energy level is capable of holding only a certain number of electrons:

- The first level holds up to two electrons maximum but can hold less.

- The second level holds up to eight electrons maximum but can hold less.

- The third level holds up to eight electrons maximum but can hold less.

- Further energy levels hold progressively larger numbers.

> - Protons have a + charge.
> - Electrons have a − charge.
> - Neutrons have no charge.

Because opposite charges attract each other, the negatively charged electrons are held in their orbits by the positive charge of the protons in the nucleus. In every atom the number of positively charged protons is equal to the number of negatively charged electrons, therefore the atom has no overall charge: it is electrically neutral.

> The atom is always neutral because the number of protons in the nucleus is equal to the number of electrons orbiting around the nucleus.

The arrangement of particles in an atom of oxygen

- First level has two electrons therefore is full.

- Second level has eight electrons therefore is full.

- Third level has six electrons therefore is not full (it could hold eight).

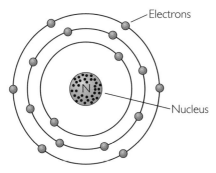

The Nucleus contains 16 protons and 16 neutrons tightly packed together. The 16 electrons move rapidly around the nucleus at distinct energy levels

Figure 4.3   The arrangements of particles in an atom of oxygen

Stable atoms have the maximum number of electrons in their outer shell.

Atoms of different elements combine by chemical reactions to form compounds. Atoms with the maximum number of electrons in their outer shell are said to be stable. They do not readily react with other elements, for example:

Helium (He) has two protons, two neutrons and two electrons.

Neon (Ne) has ten protons, ten neutrons and ten electrons.

On the other hand, some atoms contain less than the maximum number of electrons in their outer shell and are, therefore, more reactive.

Reactive atoms contain less than the maximum number of electrons in their outer shell.

Reactive atoms (see Figure 4.5 on page 80) have a great 'desire' to have the maximum number of electrons in their outer shell. In order to achieve a stable electron pattern, they are able to gain or lose electrons by reacting with other elements to form compounds. The sodium atom has one electron in its outer shell; it needs to lose this to attain a stable electron pattern

Figure 4.4   Stable atoms

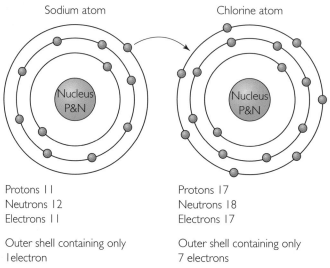

Sodium atom

Chlorine atom

Protons 11
Neutrons 12
Electrons 11

Protons 17
Neutrons 18
Electrons 17

Outer shell containing only
1 electron

Outer shell containing only
7 electrons

Figure 4.5   Reactive atoms

of eight in the outer shell. The chlorine atom has seven electrons in its outer shell; it needs to gain an electron to give the maximum eight electrons in its outer shell. Sodium and chlorine will therefore readily react together – sodium giving an electron and chlorine receiving an electron. The compound thus formed will be sodium chloride:

$$Na^+ + Cl^- \rightarrow NaCl$$

Ions

When an atom gains or loses an electron from its outer shell it becomes an ion.

When the sodium atom loses its electron from the outer shell, it will have one more proton than electrons, will have a positive charge, and will be called an

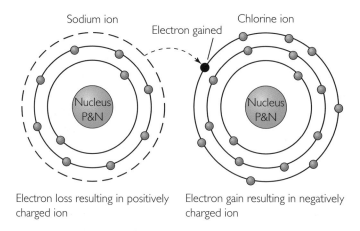

Sodium ion

Electron gained

Chlorine ion

Electron loss resulting in positively
charged ion

Electron gain resulting in negatively
charged ion

Figure 4.6   Ions

ion. A positively charged ion is called a **cation** (+).

When the chlorine atom gains an electron, it will have one more electron than protons, will have a negative charge, and will be called an ion. A negatively charged ion is called an **anion** (−).

Cations are positively charged (+).

This taking and giving of electrons will apply to all reactive atoms and the following principles also apply:

- When an atom gains or loses electrons it becomes a charged particle called an ion.

- If an atom loses electrons it becomes a positively charged ion called a cation.

- If an atom gains electrons it becomes a **negatively charged** ion called an **anion**.
  (This is easy to remember by taking the first two letters of *an*ion giving a negative ion.)

Anions are negatively charged (−).

A N I O N

A N egative ION

Ions react with each other according to definite laws:

- Ions with the same charge repel (move away from each other).

- Ions with the opposite charge will attract (move towards each other).

(Remember this as it is the fundamental principle on which some galvanic treatments work.)

Electricity

Electricity is the movement of electrons from one atom to another. It may be static or dynamic. Electricity can be produced in three ways:

1 Static electricity produced by friction.

2 Current or dynamic electricity produced by chemical reactions.

3 Current or dynamic electricity produced by magnetic fields.

Static electricity

Certain substances when rubbed together produce electrical charges or static electricity. The electrons from one material can be transferred to the other material. The material losing electrons becomes positively charged, while the one gaining electrons becomes negatively charged. Remember, these charges obey certain laws of physics: like charges repel each other, while opposite charges attract each other.

This can be demonstrated when brushing hair. The friction of brushing removes electrons from the atoms of the hair. These electrons collect on the brush giving it a negative charge. Loss of electrons leave the hair with a positive charge. Since like charges repel and opposite charges attract, the hairs will fly apart, but will be attracted to the brush. Small crackling noises will be heard and sparks seen in the dark as energy is released.

> Electric current is a flow of free electrons through a material called a conductor.

Current electricity

An electric current is a flow of free electrons through a material called a conductor; it flows from an area of excess of electrons to an area of deficiency. In order to achieve current flow a potential difference (PD) or electric force must exist between two ends of the conductor. This force is measured in volts. Some materials, such as metals, are good conductors of electrical charge. This is because the electrons in their outer shell are weakly held to their atoms and can easily be made to flow through the material (Figure 4.7).

> Electric current flows from an area of excess of electrons to an area of deficiency.

In other materials, the electrons are firmly held to their atoms, are reluctant to be detached and cannot be made to flow through the material. These are non-conductors or insulators. All materials offer some resistance or impedance to the flow of current.

> The potential difference is the force required to keep the electrons flowing; it is measured in volts.

As previously stated, the flow of electrons through the conductor requires a potential difference (PD) to exist between the ends of the wire. This is sometimes called the electronic force (EMF) and is measured in **volts**. The greater the force, the greater the intensity of the current. This force can be provided by chemical reactions in

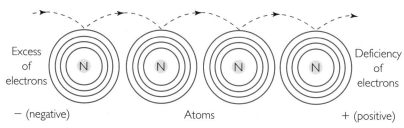

Figure 4.7   Electrons flowing through a length of wire

batteries or cells; or by using magnetic fields in generators.

Examples of conductors and insulators	
Conductors*	Insulators+
Copper	Rubber
Zinc	Plastic
Carbon	Glass
Brass	Dry wood

*Good conductors are materials whose electrons are weakly held to their atoms and can easily be made to flow through the material.

+Insulators have electrons that are firmly held to their atoms and cannot flow through the material.

A conductor is a material through which an electric current flows.

Production of electricity by chemical reaction

A simple cell or battery is a means of converting chemical energy into electrical energy. When two different metals called electrodes are immersed in a chemical called an electrolyte, an electric current is produced. The electrolyte is a chemical compound which dissociates into ions when dissolved in water. These ions move towards or away from the electrodes, depending upon their charge.

The metal which is higher in the activity series (in this case the zinc) becomes the negative electrode having an excess of electrons; the other electrode (in this case the carbon) becomes the positive electrode having a deficiency of electrons. Therefore electrons will flow through the wire from the zinc electrode to the carbon electrode. This flow of electrons will continue until all the chemicals in the electrolyte are used up, at which time the current flow will stop.

Figure 4.8 A simple cell

An electrolyte is a chemical compound which dissociates into ions and can transport an electric current.

Dry cell batteries, being easily transportable, are now widely used to power radios, torches and portable beauty therapy equipment.

The principle of how they work is the same as described above, but their construction is different. The electrolyte is a paste contained within a zinc electrode casing; the carbon rod electrode is placed down the centre. As the chemicals are used up, the battery becomes 'flat' and is disposed of.

Rechargeable batteries are available, which may be recharged by connecting them to a mains-powered battery charger. They are usually left on overnight to recharge and can then be reused when required.

Figure 4.9   Structure of a dry battery

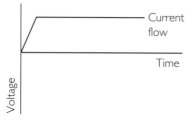

Figure 4.10   Direct current flowing in one direction

The type of current produced by cells and batteries always flows in the same direction and is called direct current (DC) or constant current.

Electricity by electro-magnetic induction

Electricity obtained from the mains is produced by a dynamo or generator in large power stations. It is produced using magnetism. When a coil of wire is rotated between the north and south poles of a magnet, it cuts through the magnetic lines of force or the magnetic field and an electromagnetic force (EMF) is produced in the coil (i.e. electrons will flow through the wire). An EMF can also be induced by moving a magnet through a coil of wire.

Each power station will have a number of these generators for producing electricity. The long coils of wire are rotated by water power or by steam from boilers heated by coal, oil or nuclear energy. Each coil of wire is rotated at speed between the poles of a large magnet.

As the coil rotates, it cuts through the lines of force each half revolution, and this produces an alternating current.

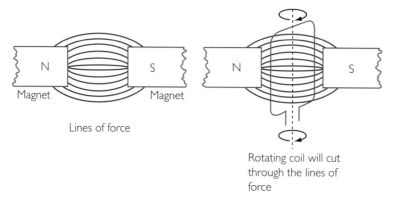

Figure 4.11   Rotating coil cutting through lines of force

Beginning at zero, the current rises to a maximum positive value, falls to zero and then rises to a maximum negative value and returns to zero with each revolution.

One complete revolution is known as a cycle. Half the cycle will rise to maximum positive and half to maximum negative. The number of these cycles produced per second is known as the frequency of the current. The unit of frequency is the **hertz** (Hz).

The frequency of the mains supply in the United Kingdom (UK) is 50 Hz (i.e. 50 cycles of current flow every second when current is switched on at the mains). A current can be made to oscillate at very high frequencies when the cycles are very close together.

The voltage produced at power stations is high at 11,000 volts. It is further increased and then reduced for mains supply to 240 volts. The mains voltage is different on the Continent.

Electrical units

As explained above:

- The pressure or force required to drive a current around a circuit is known as the potential difference (PD) or electromotive force, and is measured in **volts** often referred to as **voltage** (a voltmeter is used to measure voltage).

- The intensity of the current or rate of flow of the current is measured in **amps or amperes** (an ammeter is used to measure amperage).

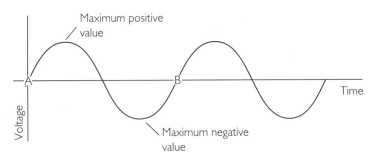

Figure 4.12   Alternating current reversing each half-cycle

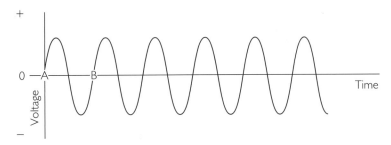

Figure 4.13   Alternating current of higher frequency

- Any conductor offers resistance to a current passing along it; this resistance is measured in **ohms**. (The longer the length of conductor, the greater the resistance. The thinner the conductor, the greater the resistance.)

The intensity of the current

The intensity of a current is the number of electrons (amps) passing one point in one second. It depends on two factors:

1   The potential difference, that is the amount of force (volts).

2   The resistance offered to the current (ohms).

The relationship between current flow (amps), potential difference (volts) and resistance (ohms) is expressed by Ohm's law.

Ohm's law

Ohm's law states that the current flowing through a circuit varies in direct proportion to the potential difference and in inverse proportion to the resistance. That is:

$$\text{current (amps)} = \frac{\text{potential difference (volts)}}{\text{resistance (ohms)}}$$

or

$$I = \frac{V}{R}$$

This means that if the PD increases, the current increases, but if the resistance increases, the current decreases. Using this formula, it is possible to calculate any one unit providing the other two are known.

Example: if the voltage is 200 volts and the resistance is 40 ohms, calculate the current.

I is the current in amps.

V is the potential difference or voltage measured in volts.

R is the resistance measured in ohms.

$$I = \frac{V}{R}$$

$$I = \frac{200}{40}$$

$$I = 50 \text{ amps}$$

Or, if the resistance is 40 ohms and the current is 50 amps, calculate the voltage.

$$V = I \times R$$

$$V = 50 \times 40$$

$$V = 200 \text{ volts}$$

Or, if the current is 50 amps and the voltage is 200 volts, calculate the resistance.

$$R = \frac{V}{I}$$

$$R = \frac{200}{50}$$

$$R = 40 \text{ amps}$$

It is easier to remember the formula by drawing a triangle:

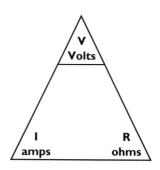

$$amps = \frac{volts}{ohms}$$

$$volts = amps \times ohms$$

$$ohms = \frac{volts}{amps}$$

Cover one unit and the other side of the equation is given by the position of the other two units.

Power

The power used when running electrical equipment is measured in watts.

$$power = current \times voltage$$

or

$$watts = amps \times volts$$

Example: the power supplied by a socket, 15 amps × 240 volts will be:

$$watts = 15 \times 240 = 3600 \text{ watts}$$
(1000 watts is 1 kilowatt)

Cost of electricity

The power of an appliance and the time for which it is used determines the amount of electricity used by that appliance. This quantity is measured in kilowatt-hours (kWh). (A kW appliance running for 1 hour uses 1 kilowatt-hour.)

The Electricity Board charges a fixed amount for each kilowatt-hour, which are known as units of electricity used. The number of units used by a house or salon

are registered on an electric meter which forms part of the mains circuit. Older meters consist of four dials which register thousands, hundreds, tens and units, but the more modern meters have a digital display showing the number of units used.

The cost of electricity is calculated by reading the meter and multiplying the number of units used by the cost per unit:

$$\text{Cost of electricity} = \text{cost per unit} \times \frac{\text{number of units}}{\text{(number of kilowatt hours)}}$$

Circuits

A circuit is the pathway taken by an electric current.

The pathway taken by an electric current is known as a circuit. In order for the current to flow, this pathway must be complete from one terminal of the electrical source to the other. If it is broken, the current flow will stop.

A closed circuit is an unbroken pathway around which the current flows continuously.

A **closed circuit** is an unbroken pathway between the negative and positive terminals of an electrical source. The current flows continuously in a closed circuit.

An **open circuit** is a pathway which is broken or interrupted by a switch or other device. This breaks the connection and stops the flow of current.

An open circuit is a broken or interrupted pathway which stops the flow of current.

A short circuit occurs when the current does not pass around its designated course but takes a short cut through a path of least resistance, for example, across a break in insulation.

A short circuit occurs when a current does not flow around the circuit but takes a path of least resistance.

Components or devices used in circuits to modify (change) currents

It is necessary to modify currents used in beauty therapy equipment. Batteries do not supply direct current (DC) at a high enough voltage for all treatment purposes, therefore mains current (AC) is used and modified.

Transformer

A transformer is a device for altering the voltage in alternating current circuits. The voltage may be increased using a step up transformer or the voltage may be decreased using a step down transformer.

A transformer is made of a soft iron core and two coils of wire. The current flows in through the primary coil and out via the secondary coil. If there are a greater number of coils in the secondary wire, the voltage will be stepped up. If there are fewer coils, the voltage will be stepped down.

REMEMBER! 'TV':
Transformer changes Voltage.

Rectifier

A rectifier is a device for changing alternating current to direct current. This process is called rectification. There are two types of rectifier:

1 A half wave rectifier: this blocks impulses in one direction.

2 A full wave rectifier: this blocks but redirects impulses in one direction.

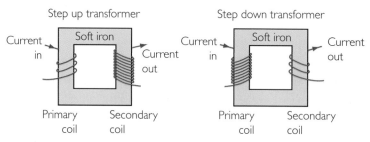

Figure 4.14   Step up and step down transformers

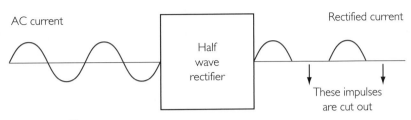

Figure 4.15   Half wave rectifier

Figure 4.16   Full wave rectifier

Capacitor or condenser

A capacitor is a device which stores electrical charge and discharges it when required. It is used to smooth the impulse pattern after rectification.

Rheostat or variable resistance

A rheostat is a device used to control the amount of current flowing through a circuit. It varies the resistance: the higher the resistance, the weaker the current. It is made of a coil of resistance wire with a sliding contact. It is wired in series with the apparatus.

If all the resistance wire is included in the circuit (contact at point B), the current will be at its lowest. The current can be increased by moving the contact towards point A. Used in wax pots to control the temperature for melting the wax and in lamps to control the intensity of light.

Figure 4.18   A rheostat

Figure 4.17   A capacitor or condenser

Potentiometer

A potentiometer is a device for varying the voltage in a circuit. It must be wired in parallel to the circuit, and is used in constant current galvanic machines to control the current during galvanic treatments.

Starter or switch

A switch or starter is a device for switching on a current, that is, starting the flow of electrons. When the client is correctly attached to the apparatus, closing the switch completes the circuit and the current will flow; when the switch is open, the circuit is broken and the current stops.

Figure 4.19   A power station

Devices used in circuits to modify currents

Device	Function	Effect
Transformer	Alters the voltage	Step up or step down
Rectifier	Changes AC to DC	Half wave or full wave
Capacitor	Stores electrical charge and discharges it as required	Smooths the impulse pattern
Rheostat	Controls the amount of current flowing through a circuit	Can increase or decrease the current
Potentiometer	Varies the voltage in a circuit	Current increases as voltage increases Current decreases as voltage decreases
Switch	Turns the current on or off	Makes or breaks the circuit

Electricity Supply

Electricity is generated in large power stations at 11,000 volts. It is more efficient to transmit electricity at even higher voltages, and transformers are used to step up the voltage to 400,000 volts. This is transmitted to substations by high-voltage cables suspended on pylons. At the substations more transformers are used to step down the voltage to suit the requirements of factories, etc., and to supply private homes and salons with a voltage of 240 volts.

Mains circuit

Electricity is supplied to the home via a cable that contains two wires – one live and one neutral – which is earthed at the substation. The mains cable enters the house and passes to a sealed box where the live wire is connected to a fuse. This box can only be opened by engineers from the Electricity Board who must investigate any faults if the fuse should 'blow'.

The mains cable then enters the meter, which registers all the units of electricity used over a period of time. It then enters the fuse box called the consumer unit. This box contains the master switch, fuses and circuit-breakers for the ring circuit, lighting circuit and others, such as for the immersion heater or cooker. If a fault develops within a circuit, the connected fuse will blow and the current flow will stop. This prevents the wire from over-heating and causing fires.

Each appliance is connected to the mains circuit sockets by a flex and a plug. This plug also contains a fuse, which is designed to blow if there is electrical over-load or if an appliance develops an electrical fault. When this fuse breaks the circuit, the appliance is effectively disconnected from the mains, but other appliances are not affected.

Fuses

A fuse is a safety device to stop the flow of electricity. It is the weakest point in a circuit. Fuses are found in the consumer unit (fuse box) and in the plugs which

Figure 4.20 Ring-main circuit

connect appliances to the mains. If a circuit is overloaded, or if the wiring or the appliance is faulty, the fuse will blow – the wire melts, breaks the circuit and the flow of electricity stops. There are two types of fuse:

Rewirable fuses

These are made of short lengths of tinned copper wire held by screws in a porcelain container. They are found in older fuse boxes. Each fuse holder is colour coded with a spot to indicate the current rating of the wire. This type of fuse is rarely found nowadays but has been included in case you have to deal with one.

Cartridge fuses

These are made of short lengths of tinned copper embedded in sand and contained in a small porcelain or glass tube. The wire is attached to metal caps at each end of the tube. In the fuse box the cartridge is housed in a metal or plastic holder. In the same way as rewirable fuses, these are colour coded to indicate the current rating. It is impossible to fit the wrong cartridge into a holder as each rating is different in size – the higher the rating the larger the cartridge.

To replace a blown fuse, first switch off the mains switch in the fuse box (this

Current ratings for various circuits		
Circuit	Current rating	Colour coding
Lighting	5A	white
Immersion heater	15A	blue
Storage heaters	20A	yellow
Ring main	30A	red
Instant hot water heater	45A	green

must be done to stop the flow of electricity to the premises and make sure that there is no chance of the operator receiving an electric shock which can prove fatal). Disconnect all appliances and check each holder in the fuse box to locate the blown fuse. Then check the relevant appliance to find the cause of the fuse blowing. It may be a fault in the appliance, such as a loose connection, a break in insulation or old, corroded fuse wire. If it is a rewirable fuse, remove the old wire and replace it with a new wire of the same current rating. If it is a cartridge fuse, remove and discard the old fuse and replace it with a new cartridge of the same size and current rating. If a fuse continues to blow, call in an electrician to check the circuit.

Plug fuses

These are cartridge-type fuses that are fitted on to the live wire in the plug and are designed to protect the appliance. Plug cartridge fuses are all the same size but they have three different current ratings:

- 3A rating for use with appliances up to 700 watts.

Figure 4.21   Structure of a cartridge fuse

- 5A rating for use with appliances between 700 and 1000 watts.

- 13A rating for use with appliances between 1000 and 3000 watts.

To replace a plug fuse, disconnect the plug from the socket. Open the plug by undoing the main screw. Remove the old cartridge and replace it with a cartridge of the same rating.

Circuit-breakers

These are modern devices designed to break the circuit if a fault is present. They may be trip switches or buttons that are designed to switch to the 'off' or 'open position' if the circuit is overloaded or faulty. The circuit-breaker can easily be reset after the fault has been found and repaired. This is done by pushing the button or moving the switch.

> Fuses/circuit-breakers are designed to break the circuit and stop the flow of current. They are safety devices to protect the user from shock and to protect the equipment.

Wiring a plug

Unscrew and remove the cover, and then examine the plug. There are three connector terminals connecting with each pin that are labelled:

E for earth
L for live
N for neutral

Figure 4.22   Wiring a plug

Across the live terminal is the fuse and at the base of the plug is a cord grip.

Next examine the flex: this is insulated with a thick outer layer of rubber or plastic. Inside are three wires with coloured insulating covers. The wires in new flexes have different colour coding from the wires in old flexes. The wires should be connected as follows:

How the wires should be connected		
Terminal	Colour	Old colour coding
E (earth)	green and yellow	green
L (live)	brown	red
N (neutral)	blue	black

Cut back the outer insulation to expose around 4 cm of the inner wires, and then cut the insulation around each wire exposing just over 1 cm of wire at the end – twist the bare wire around. Push the flex under the cord grip and screw the grip down (make sure that the grip holds the insulation) and bend each wire towards the correct terminal. The terminal may have a hole and a screw clamp or may require the wire to be placed around a post and then screwed down. Bend the end of the wire and push it into the hole or twist it in a clockwise direction around the post, and then screw tightly. Make sure that the wires are just the right length to reach their terminals without strain. The insulation should reach the screw. Check that the correct colour wires have been connected to the appropriate terminals. It is most important to connect the earth wire securely as this is a safety device. Should the casing become 'live', the earth wire conducts the current safely to earth, thus preventing a shock if the appliance is touched.

Replace the fuse checking that it is the correct size. Screw the cord grip tightly, replace the cover and screw down tightly.

If an appliance has only two wires, a live and neutral, which are connected to the appropriate L and N terminals, it is still safe to use because manufacturers have ensured that the appliance is double insulated so that no electricity can pass to the user even if there is a fault. These appliances will show the symbol ▣ indicating that it is double insulated.

Sockets

In order to provide the appliance with electricity, the plug must be pushed firmly into the socket and switched on. The socket has three rectangular holes and a switch; the live and neutral holes have shutters. The earth pin on the plug is longer than the other pins – as this is pushed in the shutters move and the other pins can be pushed home. This is a safety device to prevent young children putting fingers or other articles into the live and neutral holes and receiving shocks which could prove to be fatal.

Electrolysis

This involves the passage of direct current through a solution which results in the production of certain chemical reactions. Some chemical compounds dissolve in water to form a solution. When the compounds dissolve, they dissociate (i.e. split) into ions; either cations (+) or anions (−). These ions increase the conductivity of the solution enabling an electric current to flow easily (a solution that conducts a current is called an electrolyte).

If direct current is made to flow through such a solution, the ions will move towards the electrode with the opposite charge because like charges repel and opposite charges attract.

- The negatively charged electrode is called the **cathode**.
- The positively charged electrode is called the **anode**.

When the current is switched on, opposite charges will attract, therefore:

- The cations (+) will move towards the cathode (−). This is known as **cataphoresis**.

■ The anions (−) will move towards the anode (+). This is known as **anaphoresis**.

Anode (+)

Cathode (−)

Region where sodium hydroxide is produced

Electrolyte

Chloride ion

Sodium ion

Figure 4.23   Electrolysis of sodium chloride solution

The chemical reactions at these electrodes will depend upon the chemical composition of the electrolyte and the electrodes.

> An electrolyte is a chemical compound which dissociates into ions and can carry an electric current.

Electrical Currents Used in Beauty Therapy

Galvanic current

A direct current is used in galvanic treatments and also for epilation. The direct current flows in one direction only and has polarity. When the current is flowing, one electrode will always be negatively charged (the cathode); the other will be positively charged (the anode). The treatments using direct current are:

■ facial treatments

   disincrustation and iontophoresis
■ body treatments

   body galvanism and iontophoresis.

High-frequency current

This is a high-frequency alternating current of around 250,000 Hz used to improve the condition of the skin.

There are two methods of application:

■ the direct method
■ the indirect method or Viennese massage.

Muscle stimulating currents

An interrupted direct current is usually used to produce currents of sufficient intensity and duration to stimulate motor nerves and produce contraction of muscles. The current may be modified low-frequency alternating current or more usually, modified direct current. A variety of pulses can be produced – these are arranged in 'trains' with rest periods in between. When the current flows, the muscle contracts; when the current stops, the muscle relaxes – this simulates normal movement.

Microcurrents

These are very low amperage modified direct current measured in microamps

1 amp = 1000 milliamps
1 milliamp = 1000 microamps

These currents produce similar effects to galvanic treatment and also can be modified to produce muscle contraction.

Interferential current

Two high-frequency alternating currents are applied diagonally to the same area of tissue. The effect on the tissue is produced by an interferential current whose frequency is the difference between the frequencies of the current applied.

Safety considerations when using electrical equipment

1 Always buy equipment from a reputable dealer, who can provide a good, reliable backup service.

2 Ensure that all equipment is regularly maintained and in good working order.

3 Ensure that insulation is sound, with no breaks or worn patches.

4 Ensure that all connections, such as leads, terminals and plugs, are sound and secure.

5 Replace fuses when necessary with those of the correct rating. If a fuse blows repeatedly, do not replace it with one of a higher rating, but seek advice from electrician.

6 Do not overload the circuit by using multiple electrical sockets.

7 Keep electrical equipment away from water. Take particular care if pads have to be moistened with water, and do not allow water to drip over the machine.

8 Do not touch electrical equipment or leads, plugs, etc., with wet hands.

9 Make sure the equipment is stable and not in a position where it may easily be pushed or topple over.

10 Ensure that flexes do not trail over the working area.

11 Always test the current on yourself before applying it to the client.

12 Cover equipment when not in use to keep free from dust.

13 Remove any faulty equipment from the working area and label it clearly with: FAULTY – DO NOT USE.

SUMMARY

States of matter

- The three states of matter are: **solid**, **liquid** and **gas**.
- All matter can exist in any one of these states, depending upon temperature and pressure.

summary continues overleaf

summary continued from previous page

Differences between the three states of matter:

Solid – particles are tightly packed, move very slightly, very dense (e.g. ice).

Liquid – particles more widely spaced, move more freely, medium density (e.g. water).

Gas – particles widely spaced, move randomly at high speed, low density (e.g. steam).

Elements

- Matter is made up of chemical elements.
- An **element** is a substance in its simplest form – it cannot be further broken down by chemical reaction.
- There are 109 known elements.
- Examples include oxygen, carbon, copper, iron.

Compounds

- A **compound** is formed when elements react and combine together to form a new substance.

Atoms

- An **atom** is the smallest part of an element which retains its distinct chemical properties and which can take part in a chemical reaction.
- An atom has a nucleus containing protons with a positive charge, and neutrons with no charge. Electrons with a negative charge orbit around the nucleus at different energy levels.
- The atom is neutral (it has no charge) because it has an equal number of protons (+) and electrons (−).

Definitions

- **Protons** are **positively** charged, found in the nucleus of an atom.
- **Neutrons** are **neutral** (i.e. have no charge), found in the nucleus of an atom.
- **Electrons** are **negatively** charged, found orbiting the nucleus at different energy levels. There are up to two electrons in the first level, and up to eight in the second and third levels, etc.
- All the atoms of an element are identical, having the same number of neutrons, protons and electrons.
- Elements are different from each other because of the different numbers of protons, electrons and neutrons in their atoms.

summary continues overleaf

summary continued from previous page

Ions

- When atoms gain or lose electrons from their outer shell/energy level, they become ions.
- If an atom **loses** electrons, it becomes a **positively** charged ion called a **cation**.
- If an atom **gains** electrons, it becomes a **negatively** charged ion called an **anion**.

Electricity

- Electricity is the movement of electrons from one atom to another. It may be static electricity, or it may be made to move through a conductor (known as dynamic or current electricity).
- When rubbed together, substances produce static electricity, because electrons pass from one to the other.
- Dynamic electricity is produced chemically by cells and batteries, or it may be produced by magnetic fields in generators.

Current electricity

- An **electric current** is a **flow** of free electrons through a material called a **conductor**, from an area where electrons are in excess to an area deficient in electrons.
- The amount of current flowing is measured in **amps**.

Potential difference (PD) or electromotive force

- This is the force required to achieve a flow of electricity through a conductor.
- Known as **voltage**, it is measured in **volts**.

Resistance

- All conductors have a tendency to resist the flow of electrons.
- Electrical **resistance** is measured in **ohms**.
- The amount of current flowing in a circuit depends on the voltage and the resistance to the current.
- The relationship between current flow (amps), potential difference (volts) and resistance (ohms) is expressed by Ohm's law.

Ohm's law

- This states that the current flowing through a circuit varies in direct proportion to the potential difference and in inverse proportion to the resistance.

$$I = \frac{V}{R}$$

When the voltage increases the current increases, when the resistance increases the current decreases.

summary continues overleaf

summary continued from previous page

Power

- The unit of power is the watt:

    watts = amps $\times$ volts

Direct current

- Cells and batteries produce direct current (DC).
- Direct current flows in one direction only, without variation. It has polarity. One electrode will be negatively charged (the cathode) and the other will be positively charged (the anode).

Alternating current

- Generators produce alternating current (AC).
- Beginning at zero, the current rises to maximum positive value, falls to zero and then rises to maximum negative value and returns to zero. This is one cycle.
- The number of cycles per second is the frequency and is measured in hertz (Hz).
- The frequency of the UK mains is 50 Hz.
- Alternating current from the mains can be modified to provide the direct current necessary for some treatments.

Devices for modifying current

- A transformer changes voltage in AC circuits. It may be a step up transformer for increasing voltage, or a step down transformer for decreasing voltage.
- A rectifier changes AC to DC, it may be a half wave rectifier or full wave rectifier.
- A capacitor or condenser stores electrical charge and discharges it when required.
- A rheostat or variable resistance varies the current flowing in a circuit. It varies the resistance – the higher the resistance the weaker the current.
- A potentiometer varies the voltage in the circuit, it may increase the voltage thus increasing current flow or it may decrease the voltage thus reducing current flow.

Fuses

- A fuse is designed to be the weakest point in the circuit.
- It is a safety device to stop the flow of current should the circuit or appliance be faulty.
- There are two types: rewirable fuse and cartridge fuse.

Colour coding and wiring of plugs

- See page 93.

Questions

1 Explain the differences in the following: solids, liquids and gases.
2 Define the term 'element' and give two examples.
3 Draw a diagram showing the structure of an atom. Label and give the electrical charge of each particle.
4 Define the following terms:
   (a) ion
   (b) cation
   (c) anion.
5 Complete the following statements:
   (a) Ions with the same charge . . .
   (b) Ions with the opposite charge . . .
6 Give two ways in which dynamic electricity is produced.
7 Explain how electricity flows through a conductor.
8 Which of the following are good conductors of electricity:
   (a) copper
   (b) carbon
   (c) plastic
   (d) brass
   (e) glass
   (f) dry wood.
9 Explain the difference between DC and AC. Draw a simple diagram to illustrate each one.
10 Explain the meaning of the following:
   (a) high frequency current
   (b) polarity
   (c) electrodes
   (d) electrolyte.
11 State Ohm's law.
12 If the resistance in a circuit increases, what happens to the current flow?
13 If the resistance in a circuit is 30 ohms and the voltage is 240 volts, calculate the current flowing around the circuit.
14 Explain the function of the following devices in a circuit:
   (a) transformer
   (b) rectifier.
15 Explain the purpose of a fuse.
16 List the terminals found in a plug and indicate the modern colour coding of connecting wires.

Treatments

5 High Frequency Treatment

OBJECTIVES

After you have studied this chapter you will be able to:

1. Identify the terminals on the machine.

2. Identify the electrodes used for each method of application.

3. Differentiate between the effects of the direct and indirect methods of application.

4. Select the appropriate method of application to meet the needs of the client.

5. Identify the contraindications to treatment.

6. Treat the client; paying due consideration to maximum efficiency, comfort, safety and hygiene.

Figure 5.1 is a photograph of a high frequency treatment unit and the electrodes used to deliver the current to the client. As its name implies, this unit uses a high frequency current (a current which alternates at over 100,000 cycles per second is known as high frequency). The high frequency output of these units is an alternating current of around 250,000 Hz at a high voltage but low current flow. This alternating current will not stimulate muscle contraction because the duration of the pulses is too short. It passes easily through the skin to produce heating effects. High frequency is used for its thermal effects.

Figure 5.1   High frequency unit with electrodes

There are two methods of application:

1 The direct method.

2 The indirect method (Viennese massage).

These two methods have different effects on the tissues and must be selected carefully to suit the client. They are primarily used on the face but may also be used on the body – the technique, effects, etc., are similar for both.

High Frequency Equipment

Units producing high frequency currents require only two controls: an on/off switch and an intensity control. The current is delivered to the client by means of one electrode; different electrodes are used for the direct and indirect methods of application.

Electrodes used for the direct method

Figure 5.2 shows a variety of electrodes shaped for specific purposes. They are made of glass with metal end connections. A very small amount of air, neon or mercury, is sealed inside the tube. When the electrode is pushed into its holder, the metal end makes contact with a metal plate in the holder. When the current is switched on, it flows from the machine, through the holder, to the electrode. The air or gas inside the tube ionises, the current flows through the tube and is dispersed into the tissues under the electrode. The electrodes glow violet if they contain air or orange if they contain neon. If they contain mercury vapour, they will glow a blue-violet colour and give off ultraviolet rays. Most of these rays will not pass

Figure 5.2   Portable high frequency showing electrodes

through the tubes as they are made of glass, which absorbs ultraviolet radiation. A metal electrode is sometimes found inside the glass which intensifies the effect.

The electrode used for the indirect method

This is known as a saturator. It may be made of metal or glass and again fits into a holder. The client holds the holder in one hand and the saturator is held firmly in the other hand.

The current passes through the holder into the saturator and 'charges' the client. The therapist massages the client and the current is 'drawn off' through the therapist's fingers. The therapist is part of the circuit when giving this treatment.

Rings must not be worn on the hand that holds the saturator.

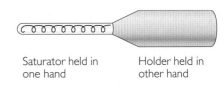

Saturator held in one hand   Holder held in other hand

Figure 5.3 Electrode used for indirect high frequency treatment

The Direct Method

This method is particularly suitable for the client with greasy, seborrhoeic, acne prone skin due to its stimulating, drying effect. It may also be used on dry and mature skin. (The treatment time for this type of skin must be short – around 5 minutes – otherwise the condition will be exacerbated.)

This method uses a glass electrode which is moved slowly over the skin; it is sometimes known as **effluvation**. The current passes from the electrode and is dispersed over the skin. The warmth generated in the tissues will produce the beneficial effects for the client. The sparking is used for its germicidal effect.

Uses

1 To dry and improve the condition of seborrhoeic skin.

2 To dry greasy skins and greasy areas on a combination skin (dry/greasy skin).

Figures 5.4 Treatment using high frequency

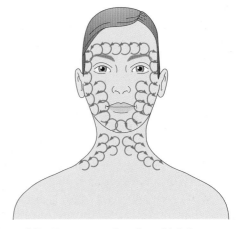

Figure 5.5 Treatment using direct high frequency

3 To improve the condition of blemished skin.

4 To destroy bacteria and aid healing of acne and pustular prone skin by means of sparking.

5 To increase sebaceous secretions on a dry, mature skin. In order to achieve this, the treatment is carried out for a short time only (4–5 minutes) and uses the warmth created by the current (too long a treatment will increase the dryness).

Effects

1 **Production of heat**. The rapidly oscillating current produces rapid motion of the molecules in the tissues which generates heat. This heating is greatest in the superficial tissues under the electrode.

2 **Increased metabolic rate**. Metabolism is a chemical reaction capable of being accelerated by heat. An increase in metabolic rate creates a demand for oxygen and nutrients and an increase in output of waste products. This promotes healing and improves the condition of the skin.

3 **Vasodilation resulting in hyperaemia and erythema**. Heat causes vasodilation and an increase in the flow of blood to the area. The increase in metabolism produces an increase in metabolites which act on capillary walls producing dilation; this also increases the blood supply. In this way, oxygen and nutrients are brought more rapidly to the area and waste products are carried away. This improves the condition of the skin.

4 **Soothing effects on nerves**. Mild heat has a soothing effect on nerve endings, producing a feeling of relaxation.

5 **Increased activity of sebaceous glands**. Warmth increases the activity of sebaceous glands. This aids the release of blockages caused by build up of sebum. It increases the lubrication of dry, dehydrated skins.

6 **Germicidal effect**. When the electrode is held just off the skin (no more than 7 mm or ¼ inch away), the current jumps across the gap forming a spark. The oxygen in the air is ionized and forms ozone, which destroys bacteria and promotes the healing of papules and pustules. As the current jumps, the spark produces ultraviolet rays, which destroy bacteria. The sparking itself may burn and destroy bacteria. Great care must be taken when sparking as too large a gap and too long a spark can destroy the tissues.

This effect can be used medically for the removal of warts, skin tags, etc. It is known as **fulguration**.

7 **Drying effects**. The sparks stimulate nerve endings in the skin, which result in the constricting of the pores. Oxygen in the air is converted to ozone, which has a drying effect.

Sparking must be done with care. No more than 7 mm/¼ inch away for 1–2 secs.

Contraindications

1 Cuts and abrasions.

2 Vascular conditions and hypersensitive skins.

3 Hairy areas.

4 Metal fillings (excessive) or heavy bridge work.

5 Sinus blockages.

6 Tense, nervous clients upset by the noise of the machine.

7 Skin disorders/diseases, infections.

8 Sunburn.

Dangers

1 The main danger/risk with high frequency current is shock. Shock may be caused in the following ways:
   (a) Touching faulty apparatus.
   (b) Wearing jewellery during treatment.
   (c) Touching metal objects which earths the current.
   (d) Lifting the electrode off the skin during treatment.
   (e) Placing the electrode on the skin after the intensity is turned up and lifting it off the skin before the intensity is turned down.

2 Destruction of tissues if sparking is at too great a distance and for too long a time.

Precautions

1 Remove all metal and jewellery from the treatment area.

2 Ensure that the client is not touching any metal, such as the frame of the couch.

3 Warn the client of the machine's noise and explain the treatment.

4 Always keep the electrode in contact with the client.

5 Do not use skin lotions containing alcohol as alcohol is highly flammable (although the danger of igniting it is extremely small).

6 Do not spark more than 7 mm (¼ inch) away from the skin surface as this is destructive to tissues.

7 Speak to the client during the treatment, ensure her comfort and be alert to contra-actions.

Treatment technique

Preparation of the client

1 Place the client in a well-supported and comfortable position.

2 Check that all jewellery has been removed.

3 Check for contraindications.

4 Explain the treatment to the client, tell her of the noise produced by the machine and reassure her as necessary.

5 Cleanse the skin but do not use a toner containing alcohol.

6 Apply talc or ozone cream to the face and neck to facilitate movement of

the electrode, or apply a clean gauze rectangle.

Procedure

1 Place the machine on a suitable, stable base and check the plugs and leads.

2 Check the intensity control is at zero.

3 Collect all commodities.

4 Test the machine.

5 Select a suitable electrode and clean it with a disinfectant wipe.

6 Place the electrode on the client's face, switch on the machine and increase the intensity up to the client's tolerance. This may have to be decreased over bony areas. The therapist's free hand should rest on the pillow or hold the cable. Do not place on the client's face as it will draw off the current or produce a mild electric shock if moved on and off.

7 Massage in broad circular movements over the face and neck without breaking contact with the skin. The more superficial the movement, the greater the stimulation.

8 Spark if necessary (the electrode may need changing).

9 Lower the intensity to zero and switch off the machine before removing the electrode from the client's face.

10 Remove the medium and tone the skin.

11 Clean the electrode carefully by wiping with hot water and detergent and then a disinfectant wipe. Take particular care not to wet the metal contact.

Timing of treatments

■ Oily skin: 10–15 minutes

■ Dry, dehydrated skin: 3–5 minutes

REMEMBER! Feedback and after care.

The Indirect Method or Viennese Massage

This method is used for clients with dry, lined and dehydrated skin. This method uses a saturator which is held firmly in the client's hand. The holder is held in the other hand (see Figure 5.3). When the current is switched on, it flows through the saturator and charges the client; the therapist massages the client's face and the current discharges from the face to the massaging fingers. The therapist is part of the circuit during indirect high frequency treatments. This is a warming and relaxing treatment.

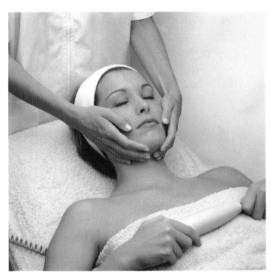

Figure 5.6   Treatment with indirect high frequency

Figure 5.7   Treatment with indirect high frequency

Uses

1 To improve the condition of dry, dehydrated skin.
2 To improve sluggish circulation.
3 To improve the condition of tired skin with fine lines.
4 To promote the relaxation of tissues.

Effects

1 Warmth is produced in the superficial tissues.
2 Vasodilation of surface capillaries producing hyperaemia and erythema.
3 The increase in blood flow to the area will bring nutrients and oxygen to nourish the tissues and will remove waste products. This will improve the condition of tissues.
4 The increase in metabolic rate due to heating will also improve the condition of the skin.

5 The mild warmth and slow massage has a sedative effect on the sensory nerve endings and produces relaxation of the tissues.
6 The friction produced by the massage movements aids desquamation (loss of dead skin).
7 Stimulates sebaceous glands.

Contraindications

1 Hypersensitive skin.
2 Vascular conditions.
3 Cuts and abrasions.
4 Skin diseases/disorders, infections.
5 Sunburn.

Dangers

Shock as for direct high frequency treatment. (See page 107)

Precautions

1 Remove all jewellery and metal. If the client is unable or unwilling to remove a wedding ring, the holder can be held in the ringed hand and the saturator in the hand free of jewellery.

2 Ensure that the client is not touching any metal.

3 Warn the client of the noise from the machine.

4 The client must be told to hold the saturator firmly – one hand holding the holder and the other holding the saturator firmly (sparks will occur if the saturator is loosely held).

5 Put talc on the hand.

6 Always keep one hand in contact with the client when turning the machine on and off. Remember that removing one hand from the face intensifies the current through the other hand, and avoid creating discomfort especially over bony areas, such as the forehead.

7 Speak to the client during the treatment.

Treatment technique

Preparation of the client

1 Place the client in a well-supported and comfortable position.

2 Check that all jewellery has been removed.

3 Check for contraindications.

4 Explain the treatment to the client, tell her of the noise produced by the machine and reassure her as necessary.

5 Cleanse the skin.

6 Apply talc to the face and neck for a superficial and more stimulating effect. Apply cream for a soothing, relaxing effect.

Procedure

1 Place the unit on a suitable, stable base and check all plugs and leads.

2 Check that the intensity controls are at zero.

3 Collect all commodities.

4 Test the machine.

5 Wipe the saturator with a disinfectant wipe and ask the client to hold the saturator firmly. If necessary, talc the hand to absorb any perspiration.

6 Place one hand on the client's face and, using small circular movements, begin to massage the area.

7 Turn the machine up slowly within the client's tolerance.

8 Place the other hand on the opposite side of the face and massage slowly with both hands. Warmth should be felt in the fingers.

9 Do not lose contact with both hands as this will result in a shock to the client.

10 At the end of the treatment, remove one hand from the client's face, reduce the current intensity slowly to zero and switch off the machine.

11 Remove the cream or talc.

12 Clean the saturator carefully by wiping with hot water and detergent and then with a disinfectant wipe. Take particular care not to wet the metal contact.

Timing of treatment

Apply for 8–20 minutes, depending on client's skin type, skin reaction and client tolerance.

REMEMBER! Feedback and after care.

SUMMARY

- A high frequency current is a rapidly oscillating current of over 100,000 Hz (cycles per second).
- The frequency produced by beauty therapy equipment is around 250,000Hz.
- It passes easily through the skin to produce heating effects.
- It will not stimulate muscles to contract as the frequency is too high and, therefore, the pulse duration is too short.
- High frequency current may be applied to the body in two ways: the direct method and the indirect method (Viennese massage).

The direct method

- With the direct method, the current is applied to the skin by means of a glass electrode. It is used for its warming and stimulating effects. Sparking is used for its germicidal effect. Sparking must be carried out with care, it must be done quickly and the gap between the electrode and the skin should be less than 7 mm or ¼ inch. If sparking is done slowly and with too big a gap, the tissues may be destroyed.
- Skin types that benefit from direct high frequency treatment are: greasy seborrhoeic skin; blemished skin with papules and pustules; a sluggish skin; it may be used on dry, mature skin to stimulate activity in sebaceous glands, but this must only be done for a short time (4–5 minutes).
- The treatment time for oily skin is 10–15 minutes.

The indirect method

- With the indirect method, the current is carried to the client via a saturator electrode which is held in the client's hand. The current is then 'drawn off' through the fingers of the therapist massaging the skin. The therapist forms part of the circuit for the indirect method.
- It is used for its warming and relaxing effect.

summary continues overleaf

summary continued from previous page

- Skin types that benefit from indirect high frequency are: dry, dehydrated skin; sluggish skin; mature, tired skin with fine lines.
- The treatment time is 8–20 minutes depending upon the skin type and client tolerance.

Dangers of high frequency treatments

- Shock because of the easy discharge of the current. Ensure that the client removes all metal jewellery and that she cannot accidentally touch metal objects, such as trolleys and bed frames.
- The destruction of tissues through sparking when using the direct method. Sparking must be done quickly over a pustule, with less than a 7 mm gap (¼ inch) from the surface of the skin.

QUESTIONS

1   Explain what is meant by a high frequency current.
2   Give two different methods of application.
3   List the skin types which would benefit from each method.
4   Explain what is meant by 'sparking'.
5   When would sparking be used and at what distance?
6   How does sparking produce its effect?
7   List the contraindications to direct high frequency treatment.
8   Explain why the electrode must be and remain in contact with the skin when the current is switched on and off.
9   Which method is most suitable for the tense client with mature, dry skin?
10 Why is the therapist said to be part of the circuit in the indirect method?
11 Give the main dangers to the client when using high frequency treatment.
12 Explain the procedure for cleaning the electrodes after use.

Oral questions

Direct high frequency

1   Name the type of current used in high frequency treatments.
2   Why is this treatment suitable for a client with greasy, seborrhoeic skin?

questions continues overleaf

questions continued from previous page

3   What is meant by the term 'germicidial effect'?

4   How does direct high frequency produce its germicidial effect?

5   Why would you instruct the client to remove jewellery?

6   Is direct high frequency a suitable treatment for mature skin?

7   Why would you not use a toner containing alcohol prior to the treatment?

8   What is a safe distance for sparking?

9   Why does sparking destroy tissues?

10   Where should the therapist's free hand be placed and why?

11   How do you gain feedback from the client after treatment?

12   How would you clean the electrode after treatment?

13   Why is the use of talc not recommended as a medium for the treatment?

Indirect high frequency

1   What does high frequency current mean?

2   Why is this treatment called indirect high frequency?

3   Why is this treatment suitable for clients with dry, lined, dehydrated skin?

4   What do you understand by metabolic rate of the cells?

5   What would happen if you removed both hands from the client's skin before turning the current off?

6   Why did you apply cream to the face before starting the treatment?

7   Would you use any other type of medium?

8   What are the approximate timings of this treatment?

9   When may you need to stop the treatment?

10   Why is it important to ensure that the client places her hands on top of the cover during treatment?

6 Mechanical Massage

After you have studied this chapter you will be able to:

1 Distinguish between the different types of mechanical massage equipment.

2 Distinguish between the effects produced by the different types of equipment and the various 'heads'.

3 Select the appropriate massage equipment to suit the needs of the client.

4 Identify any contraindications to the treatment.

5 Treat the client, paying due consideration to maximum efficiency, comfort, safety and hygiene.

Figure 6.1 is a photograph of just one type of equipment used for mechanical massage. Mechanical massage is the manipulation of body tissues using machines. Generally, mechanical massage is used in conjunction with other treatments to relieve muscle tension and muscle pain, to improve the circulation and to improve certain skin conditions. Providing the client is on a reducing diet, the heavier vibrations may help to disperse fatty deposits from specific areas of the body.

Many different types of appliances are manufactured to produce effects similar to those of a manual massage. They vary from the small hand-held percussion and audiosonic equipment designed to treat small, localized areas, to the large, heavy gyratory massagers used for deeper effects on large areas of the body. Although the effects are similar to those of manual massage, the sensation felt by the client is very different. The treatment is rather impersonal and the use of a machine rather than the touch of hands is not as pleasing to the client.

In practice, most mechanical massage treatments should be combined with some manual massage, thus gaining the more personal aspects of manual massage combined with the depth and power of vibratory equipment. Using mechanical massage equipment is certainly less tiring for the beauty therapist than performing a long, vigorous manual massage. The effects produced are similar for all types

Figure 6.1   A gyratory body massager

of massage equipment, but are deeper and greater with the heavier machines. The treatment is very popular with clients as they feel invigorated and consider that the desired results will be achieved.

Gyratory Massagers

Gyratory massagers are available for use on the face and the body. These appliances enable the therapist to perform a deep and thorough massage. The floor-standing gyratory massager shown in Figure 6.1, commonly called G5, provides a deep body massage.

Figure 6.2   A gyratory facial massager

Figure 6.3   Hand-held massager

The table model shown in Figure 6.2, provides a deep facial massage. There are portable hand held-body massagers available but these are heavy to use as all the electrical components are held in the hand. They do not achieve the same depth but are useful for domiciliary work. The principles of treatment are the same for all models.

Body Treatment

The floor-standing gyratory massager known as G5 includes vibration and percussion. It provides a deep, vigorous massage which is very effective and is a very popular treatment in the salon.

It has all the working electrical components housed in a box supported on a stand, only the moving head is held in the hand. A rotary electric motor turns a crank which is attached to the head. The head is driven to turn in a gyratory motion, moving round and round, up and down and side to side with pressure, providing a deep massage. A variety of attachments is available, which screw on to the head; they are designed to simulate the movements of manual massage:

- round sponge-effleurage
- curved sponge-effleurage
- disc sponge-effleurage
- hard rubber heads-petrissage
- single and double ball-petrissage
- flat disc-petrissage
- four half-ball-petrissage (eggbox)
- multi-half spike-petrissage
- fine spiky-tapotement
- brush heads-tapotement

Uses

1 For spot reduction of fatty deposits in conjunction with other treatments and reduced food intake.

2 To relieve muscular tension.

3 To reduce muscular aches and pains.

4 To improve poor circulation.

5 To improve the texture of dry, flaky, rough skin.

Effects

1 As with manual massage, the main effect is stimulation of the circulation. The movements speed up the flow of blood in the veins, removing deoxygenated blood and waste products more rapidly. This affects the arterial circulation bringing oxygenated blood and nutrients to the area. Lymph drainage via the lymphatic vessels is also increased.

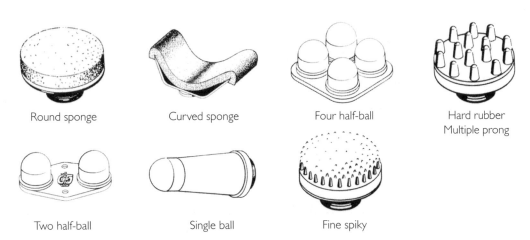

Round sponge   Curved sponge   Four half-ball   Hard rubber Multiple prong

Two half-ball   Single ball   Fine spiky

Figure 6.4 Examples of different heads for the gyratory massager

2 Increased blood supply will increase the metabolic rate in the tissues. This will improve the condition of the tissues.

3 Increased blood supply and friction of the heads will raise the temperature of the area, thus will aid muscle relaxation and relieve pain.

4 Pain in muscles may also be relieved due to rapid removal of waste products, such as lactic acid.

5 Surface capillaries dilate giving an erythema. This improves skin tone.

6 The desquamating effect of the heads may improve the texture of the skin.

7 The continuous heavy pressure on adipose tissue and increased circulation to the area may aid the dispersion of fatty deposits if the client is on a reducing diet.

Contraindications

1 Skin diseases and disorders.

2 Bruises.

3 Dilated capillaries.

4 Varicose veins.

5 Thrombosis or phlebitis.

6 Skin tags, warts or pigmented moles.

7 Recent operations and scar tissue.

8 Treatment of the abdomen during pregnancy and menstruation.

9 Extremely hairy areas.

10 Thin, bony clients.

11 Elderly clients with thin, crêpey skin and lack of subcutaneous fat.

12 Acute back and spinal problems (e.g. disc trouble).

Dangers

Heavy and prolonged treatments can cause bruising and dilated capillaries. Damage to internal organs (do not treat the abdomen with poor muscle tone).

Precautions

1 Check for contraindications.

2 Do not use heavy petrissage or percussion over bony areas or over the abdomen with poor muscle tone.

3 Do not over treat one area, keep the head moving.

4 Keep the head surface parallel to the surface of the body and adapt to body contours.

5 Hold the head away from the client when switching on in case the head is insecure and becomes detached. Hold the head below the bed for safety.

6 Cover the heads with a plastic bag, which can be changed for each client, for hygiene reasons.

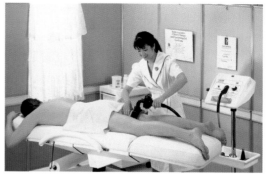

Figure 6.5   Demonstration of massage using gyratory massager

7 There are units which offer variable speeds from 20 to 60 cycles per second. Select the speed to produce the effect required: the faster the speed the more vigorous the treatment.

Treatment technique

Preparation of the client

1 Place the client in a well-supported, comfortable position.

2 Check that all jewellery has been removed.

3 Check for contraindications.

4 Clean the skin with cologne.

5 Explain the treatment to the client.

6 Select the appropriate pre-heating treatment.

7 Apply talc to the area using effleurage strokes (do not use oil as it may cause deterioration of the sponge heads).

> Hold the head away from the client when switching on to prevent injury should the head become detached.

Procedure

1 Select the appropriate heads to suit the needs of the client. Do not change the heads too often as this breaks the continuity of the treatment:
   (a) For effleurage: curved sponge on limbs or round sponge elsewhere.
   (b) For kneading: the flat disc head for lighter petrissage; the four ball head for deeper petrissage; the multi, large spike for very deep petrissage on very heavy areas of adipose tissue; single and double ball heads on specific, localized areas.
   (c) For desquamating: fine spiky and brush heads.

To maintain high standards of hygiene, the heads can be placed in a plastic bag, which should be changed for each client. Some manufacturers provide washable covers for the sponge heads.

> Apply the talcum powder sparingly and with care. Airborne particles can cause respiratory problems.

2 Switch the machine on holding the head below the level of the couch. (This is a safety precaution in case the head is insecure – if it flies off it will not hit the client.)

3 With the sponge applicator, apply in long sweeping strokes following the direction of venous return and natural contours of the body. The stroke at make and break should be light and smooth rather than abrupt and jerky. The pressure should be heavier on muscle bulk. Cover the area well.

4 Change the head for kneading. Use a circular kneading motion, using the other hand to support the tissues and lift them towards the head. Again apply upward pressure and work with venous return. Cover the area well.

Bruising can be caused by over treating, heavy use, or pressure from the hard edge of the head.

5   Keep the surface of the attachment parallel to the surface of the body at all times. (If one side lifts off the body, there is a danger of damaging the tissues with the hard edge of the head.)

Particular care should be taken when selecting heads for treating the abdominal wall. Abdominal organs have no bony framework for protection – their only protection is provided by the muscles and tissues of the abdominal wall. Overstretched muscles with poor tone offer less protection. This must be considered when treating the abdomen. The heavier petrissage heads should only be used on well-toned abdominal muscles with a covering of adipose tissue (e.g. the younger, overweight client).

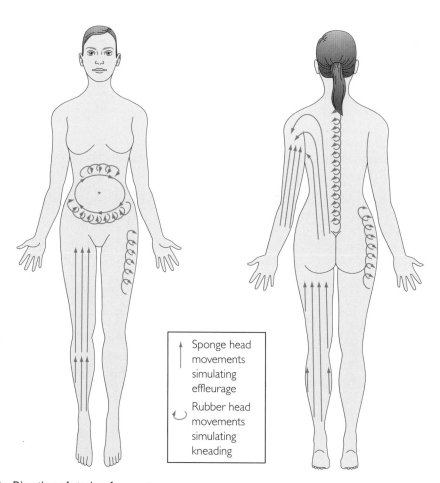

↑   Sponge head movements simulating effleurage

↻   Rubber head movements simulating kneading

Figure 6.6   Direction of strokes for gyratory massager

6 Change to the effleurage head to complete the treatment.

7 The degree of erythema and client tolerance dictates the length of the treatment.

8 Wash the heads and covers in hot water and detergent, and allow them to dry.

Percussion Vibrator

This is a hand-held appliance; it is lightweight, easy to use and to transport. As its name suggests, it is similar in effect to manual percussion movements. An electric motor is used to make the head move or tap up and down on the skin. The head can be fitted with a variety of attachments, for example, sponge or spike. Some percussion vibrators have an adjustment knob for increasing and decreasing the intensity of the tap. As the knob is tightened, the tap intensity decreases; as the knob is released the tap intensity increases. This should be carefully controlled to suit the tissues being treated. The number of movements per second is constant relating to the frequency of the current. With mains frequency of 50 Hz (cycles per second), each tap occurs every half cycle, therefore the rate of tapping will be 100 per second. Treatment time may vary from 5–15 minutes depending on the desired effects. It is used mainly on the face, neck and across the shoulders.

Uses

1 To stimulate dry, dehydrated or mature skin. The improved circulation and increase in metabolic rate will improve the condition of the skin.

2 To stimulate sebaceous glands; the warmth generated in the tissues will stimulate the production and release of sebum, which will help to lubricate dry, tired, mature skin.

3 To aid desquamation of a sluggish skin, the friction of the heads on the body part will aid the removal of the surface layer, improving texture of the skin.

4 To improve and maintain the condition of normal skin.

5 To promote relaxation of muscle fibres, the warmth produced in the area will aid relaxation and relieve

Figure 6.7   Percussion vibrator

Head

Adjustment knob

Switch

tension. It is particularly effective over localized tension nodules.

Effects

1 An increase in circulation to the treated area, bringing nutrients and oxygen to the area and removing waste products. This improves the condition of the tissues.

2 It produces vasodilation, giving hyperaemia and erythema, improving the colour and tone of the skin.

3 It increases the metabolic rate, thus improving the condition of the tissues.

4 The increase in circulation and the friction of the heads raises the temperature of the area. This promotes relaxation, relieves pain and may stimulate the activity of sebaceous glands.

5 The friction of the heads aids desquamation; this removes the surface layer of cells, improving the condition of the skin.

Contraindications

1 Any skin diseases, inflammatory disorders, chapped skin.

2 Infected acne pustules.

3 Highly vascular or telangiectic skin or dilated capillaries.

4 Sinus problems, heavy cold, fever.

5 Headaches or migraines.

6 Lean, bony features.

7 Mature skin with poor elasticity.

8 Bruises or highly sensitive skins.

Precautions

1 Check for contraindications.

2 Do not use over very bony areas.

3 Avoid the eye region.

4 Keep the head surface parallel to the surface of the face.

5 Do not overtreat one area – keep the head moving.

Audio-sonic Vibrator

This is another type of hand-held appliance. Its name is derived from the fact that the machine produces a humming sound (it should not be confused with ultrasound therapy, which is quite different). This vibrator uses an electromagnet. When the current is passing one way, the coil moves forward; as the current reverses, the coil moves back. This movement forward and backward is transmitted to the head of the appliance. When

Figure 6.8   Audio-sonic vibrator

the head is placed on the tissues, the forward–backward movement of the coil alternately compress and decompress the tissues.

Because the head does not physically move forward and backward, this appliance has a gentler action than the percussion vibrator. It penetrates more deeply into the tissues, but is less stimulating on the surface of the skin. It is, therefore, more suitable for use on sensitive areas of the face and on a mature skin. It is particularly useful for relaxing tension nodules.

Uses

Similar to the percussion vibrator.

1 To generally improve the condition of sensitive skin.

2 To stimulate dry, dehydrated, mature skin.

3 To stimulate sallow skin.

4 To aid desquamation and improve sluggish skin.

5 To produce warmth and aid relaxation of muscle fibres. Particularly effective over tension nodules.

Effects

Similar to the percussion vibrator.

1 An increase in circulation.

2 It produces vasodilation.

3 It increases the metabolic rate.

4 It raises the temperature, therefore promotes relaxation of muscle fibres and stimulates activity of sebaceous glands.

5 It aids desquamation.

Contraindications and precautions

As for percussion vibrator (page 122).

Treatment technique for percussion and audio-sonic vibrators

Preparation of the client

1 Place the client in a well-supported and comfortable position.

2 Check that all jewellery has been removed.

3 Check for contraindications.

4 Explain the treatment to the client.

5 Cleanse the skin.

6 Apply talc for oily/normal skin or cream for dry skin. (Read the manufacturer's instructions.)

Procedure

1 Select the appropriate head and secure it firmly to the vibrator.

2 Switch the machine on, away from the client.

3 Commence the treatment using straight lines or a circular motion; ensure coverage of all areas but avoid delicate areas around the eyes and prominent cheekbones.

4 The skin reaction indicates the length of the treatment time. When an even erythema is produced, the treatment should stop. This may take between 5–15 minutes.

5 The vibrator can be used indirectly over bony or sensitive areas (e.g.

cheekbones and forehead). The therapist places her hand between the face and the vibrator head. This reduces the stimulation.

6 Remove the cream and complete the facial routine.

7 Clean the heads, wash with hot water and detergent and disinfect with surgical wipes. Brushes and sponges may be soaked in disinfectant.

REMEMBER! Feedback and after care.

SUMMARY

- Mechanical massage is the manipulation of body tissues using machines.
- Types of mechanical massage equipment: gyratory massager, hand-held massager; percussion massager; audio-sonic massager.
- The hand-held massagers are used for small body and facial areas; the large massagers are used on large body areas.
- Mechanical massage is used to improve many conditions. It is usually combined with some manual massage. The client will then benefit from the personal touch and from the deeper effect of the mechanical massage.
- Mechanical massage will improve the circulation to the area, will relieve muscle tension and aches and pains, will aid the dispersal of fatty tissue in conjunction with diet and will improve the condition of the skin.
- There is little danger in application except that bruising and dilated capillaries may result from heavy or prolonged treatment.
- The head moves round and round with gyratory movement. It is used on the body.
- The percussion vibrator head moves up and down and taps on the body part. It is used on small areas, such as tension nodules, or on the face to improve the condition of the skin.
- The audio-sonic vibrator alternately compresses and decompresses the tissues due to the movement of an electromagnet within the head. Because the head does not physically tap on the area, it is much more gentle in action than the percussion vibrator. It is used on painful tension nodules and on the face to improve the condition of the skin; it is particularly suitable for sensitive skins.

Feedback
Examine the area and ask appropriate questions to obtain feedback; this will indicate if the treatment is effective and suitable and the client is happy.

After care
Give advice on immediate after care and the routine to follow before the next treatment.

QUESTIONS

1   Give three uses for mechanical massage on the body.
2   Name three different types of mechanical massage equipment.
3   List four contraindications to mechanical massage on the body.
4   List the effects of mechanical massage on the body.
5   Explain briefly why audio-sonic vibrators have an advantage over percussion vibrators on a sensitive area.
6   Give four effects of percussion vibrator treatment to the face.
7   Give two different uses for each of the following:
    (a)   gyratory massager (G5)
    (b)   percussion vibrator
    (c)   audio-sonic vibrator
8   Explain briefly how you would incorporate mechanical massage into a body treatment routine.
9   Give reasons why the heavy gyratory vibrator heads should not be used on the abdominal wall of certain clients.
10 Explain the procedure for maintaining high standards of hygiene when using gyratory massagers.

Oral questions

1   How does mechanical massage differ from manual massage?
2   Are there any advantages in using mechanical massage?
3   Are there any disadvantages in using mechanical massage?
4   Why would you use mechanical massage on a client who was overweight with hard fat and cellulite on the thighs and buttocks?
5   Why do the massage heads come in different shapes and sizes?
6   What type of condition would benefit from use of a gyratory vibrator?
7   Could you cause any harm to the client if your technique is poor?
8   How can these dangers be avoided?
9   What is happening in the tissues as you work?
10   Why did you hold the head below the couch level to switch the machine on?
11   Why did you use talc as the medium, not oil?
12   How did you protect your client from cross infection?
13   When would you use the hard spiky rubber head?

7 Vacuum Suction

OBJECTIVES

After you have studied this chapter you will be able to:

1 Identify the terminals on the machine.

2 Describe the lymphatic system.

3 Draw outlines of the face and body and indicate the positions of the main lymph nodes relevant to lymphatic drainage.

4 Identify the main lymph nodes on the human body.

5 Determine the suitability of the treatment to meet the needs of the client.

6 Describe the effects of facial and body vacuum suction.

7 Identify the contraindications to treatment.

8 Treat the client, paying due consideration to maximum efficiency, comfort, safety and hygiene.

Figure 7.1 is a photograph of a vacuum suction machine. This particular model may be used for both facial and body work, and includes a variety of cups called ventouse to suit different areas of the body. It is used to speed up the flow of lymph and blood and stimulate the metabolic rate. The treatment is based on the principle of creating reduced pressure within the cups. These are moved over the area in the direction of lymphatic drainage towards the nearest lymph nodes, into which the lymph will drain. When the pressure within the cup is reduced to below atmospheric pressure, the tissues rise into the cup. The lymphatic and blood vessels dilate as the suction is applied, and as the

Figure 7.1 A vacuum suction machine used for facial and body work

cup moves along the rate of flow will increase. Vacuum suction treatment is effective on the face and the body.

The Lymphatic System

In order to provide the most effective treatment, the therapist must have an understanding of the lymphatic system. The lymphatic system is closely associated with the blood circulatory system. It transports a fluid called lymph from the tissue spaces, and returns it to the blood via the subclavian veins. If this fluid is not drained away from tissue spaces, swelling of the area will occur – this is known as oedema.

Large protein molecules and waste products are transported via the lymphatic system back to the bloodstream. Lymphatic capillaries begin as blind end tubes and form a network throughout the tissue spaces. Their walls are very thin, allowing particles of large molecular size to pass through. Lymph capillaries join together to form larger vessels. These lymph vessels are similar to small veins in structure and have semi-lunar valves lining their walls to prevent the backward flow of lymph. All lymph vessels drain into lymph nodes. These are small, bean-shaped structures strategically placed in groups throughout the body. The lymph is filtered as it passes through each node: damaged cells, microbes, etc., are filtered and destroyed. In the nodes, lymphocytes multiply and antibodies are produced; these may be carried via the lymph into the circulation. After leaving the nodes, the lymphatic vessels join to form even larger lymph trunks. These empty into one of two lymphatic ducts:

1 **The thoracic duct** drains the whole of the body apart from the upper right quarter; it empties into the left subclavian vein.

2 **The right lymphatic duct** drains the right arm, right side of the head and chest; it empties into the right subclavian vein.

The speed at which lymph flows through the system depends on:

- The contraction and relaxation of muscles.
- The negative pressure and movement of the chest during respiration.

Backward flow of lymph is prevented by valves in the vessel walls. The volume of lymph passing into the capillaries depends on the arterial pressure and pressure of the tissue fluid.

During vacuum suction treatment, it is essential to follow the course of the lymphatic vessels and end at the nearest set of lymph nodes.

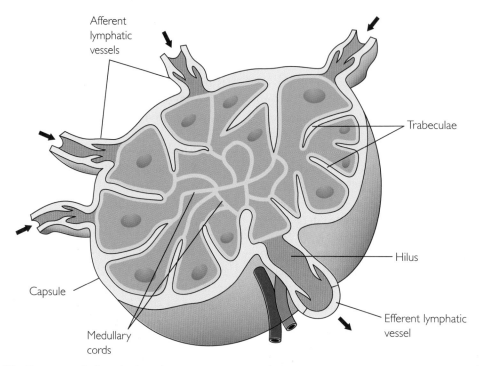

Figure 7.2 Structure of a lymphatic node

Nodes of the body and face

Body nodes	Facial nodes
Axillary nodes (in armpit)	Superficial cervical
Supratrochlear nodes (at elbow)	Deep cervical
Supraclavicular (above clavicle)	Anterior auricular (parotid)
Inguinal nodes (in groin)	Buccal
Popliteal nodes (behind knee)	Submandibular
	Submental
	Post-auricular (mastoid)
	Occipital

Vacuum Suction Units

Some of these are designed as facial units, some as body units, while others are combined units for the treatment of the face and body (see Figure 7.1). They all consist of a machine, and a selection of cups or ventouse which connect to it by plastic tubing. A suction effect is produced in the cups by sucking out air to reduce the pressure. This is done using a vacuum pump driven by an electric motor. The amount of negative pressure is registered on a gauge, and can be controlled by increasing or decreasing a regulating knob. The on/off switch controls the power from the mains. Most machines have a second outlet for blowing the air out – this can be used as a spray for a variety of preparations.

The cups are manufactured in various sizes and shapes to suit the areas of the body to be treated: small cups are for facial work and large cups are for body work. The selection of the appropriate cup to suit the body part must be carefully considered. Cups are made of glass, plastic or metal. Some cups have a small hole in the side to release the vacuum when required. This hole must be covered with a finger to maintain a vacuum (the finger is removed to release the vacuum). If there is no hole, the vacuum must be released by depressing the flesh with the finger.

Facial Vacuum Suction

Vacuum suction may be used on the face and neck for general cleansing on normal, dry, combination and greasy skins. It can be used to loosen blocked pores and blackheads (comedones) and to improve the condition of dry, dehydrated skin.

Uses

1 General skin cleansing on normal, dry, combination and greasy skins. This can be carried out following steam treatment. The time for the cleansing treatment is 5 minutes.

2 The deep cleansing of seborrhoeic skin to remove dead keratinized cells and sebum and clear follicular blockages. This is most effective following steam or disincrustation treatments to the face. The time for the treatment is 10–12 minutes.

3 To stimulate dry, dehydrated skin and improve its condition. The increased circulation, increased removal of waste products and increased cellular activity will all contribute to the improvement of the skin. The time for the treatment is 10–12 minutes.

Effects

1 It speeds up the removal of waste products via the lymphatic system.

2 It increases blood circulation to the area, bringing nutrients and oxygen, thus improving the condition of the skin.

3 It produces vasodilation giving an erythema and improving skin tone.

4 It stimulates cell metabolism.

5 It aids desquamation and the removal of dead keratinized cells, and improves the texture of the skin.

6 It loosens blockages and comedones, cleansing the pores.

Contraindications

1 Areas of telangiectasis.

2 Delicate sensitive skin.

3 Loose crêpey skin (e.g. around eyes).

4 Areas of thin skin and fine texture.

5 Infected acne.

6 Skin disorders/diseases.

7 Sunburn or windburnt skin.

Precautions

1 Select the correct cup to suit the area.

2 Check the pressure on yourself, and adjust the pressure to suit the flesh on the area being treated.

3 Apply sufficient oil to the area to facilitate the movement of the cup and provide a seal.

4 Lift enough flesh – do not exceed 20 per cent of the cup.

5 Lift the cup and move it across the contours of the face to the nearest set of lymph nodes. Do not work over the nodes.

6 Release the pressure before lifting the cup off the area.

Figure 7.3   Facial vacuum suction treatment

7 Overlap the previous stroke.

8 Do not over treat the area.

9 Speak to the client during the treatment.

Treatment technique

Preparation of the client

1 Place the client in a well-supported and comfortable position.

2 Check that all jewellery has been removed.

3 Check for contraindications.

4 Explain the treatment to the client.

5 Cleanse the skin, apply steam or disincrustation treatment.

6 Apply oil to the face and neck.

Procedure

1 Place the machine on a stable base and check the plug and leads.

2 Check that the intensity controls are at zero.

3 Collect all commodities.

4 Test the machine.

5 Wipe the cup with disinfecting fluid (e.g. surgical spirit).

6 Select the appropriate cup.

7 Place the cup on the area and adjust the suction – do not exceed 20 per cent of the ventouse. Hold it like a pencil and perpendicular to the skin.

8 Lift the cup and glide it according to the contours of the face to the nearest set of lymph nodes.

9 Break the suction before lifting the cup off the skin (use the release hole or depress the skin with the little finger).

10 Move on to the next stroke; overlap the previous stroke until the area is covered. Repeat 5–8 times depending upon the skin reaction and whether the skin is preheated. An erythema will develop more quickly if the skin is preheated.

11 Continue until the neck and face are covered. The pattern of strokes in Figure 7.5 is a guide to the drainage to named nodes in Figure 7.4.

12 Use the appropriate cup for extracting comedones and blockages or for treating wrinkles.

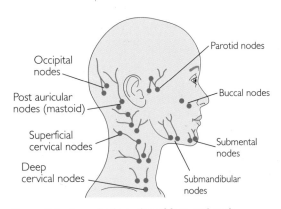

Figure 7.4 Lymphatic nodes of face and neck

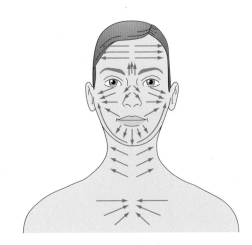

Figure 7.5 Direction of strokes for facial vacuum suction

13 Remove the oil and tone.

14 Wash the cup and tube in hot water and detergent and sterilize by soaking in disinfectant such as Milton, Cydex or Barbicide.

REMEMBER! Feedback and after care.

Body Vacuum Suction

Vacuum suction on the body is always used in conjunction with other treatments. The suction may be applied by the moving cup method or may be applied using stationary cups with a pulsating on–off vacuum.

Uses

1 To reduce fatty deposits on the abdomen, hips, thighs, dowager's hump, below the neck, etc., in conjunction with other treatments and diet.

2 To improve and reduce areas of cellulite.

3 To improve poor circulation, both lymphatic and blood.

4 To reduce non-systemic oedema and areas of fluid retention.

5 To improve the condition of the skin.

Effects

1 The flow of lymph is speeded up. As previously explained, the negative pressure inside the cup makes the tissues rise into the cup. As it does this, the vessels dilate and fill up with lymph; as the cup moves along it draws lymph with it as the vessels expand and recoil. The stroke will end just before the lymph node and lymph will drain into the node. As the flow of lymph is speeded up, more waste products will be removed.

2 Oedema may be reduced. Because the flow of lymph in the vessels is speeded up, more lymph will be drained from the tissues thus reducing stagnation and swelling. This works well for gravitational oedema but not for oedema caused by high blood pressure, kidney problems and other systemic problems. (Seek a doctor's advice to establish the cause of the oedema.)

3 Circulation is increased. In the same way as lymph vessels are affected, the veins will alternately expand and recoil and the venous flow is speeded up. If blood flows more quickly in the veins, then the arterial side may also speed up. This increases the supply of nutrients and oxygen to the body part and speeds up the removal of waste. This will improve the condition of the tissues.

4 The increased circulation will produce heat and vasodilation with erythema (this improves the colour of the skin).

5 Cell metabolism is stimulated and this improves the condition of the skin.

6 The friction of the cup, the oil used on the part and the stimulation of the circulation will aid desquamation, thus also improving the condition of the skin.

7 Venous flow is speeded up and this can help to prevent varicose veins. (If varicose veins are already present, do not use vacuum suction over the area as it will exacerbate the condition.) If varicose veins are present in the calf, the thigh can be treated.

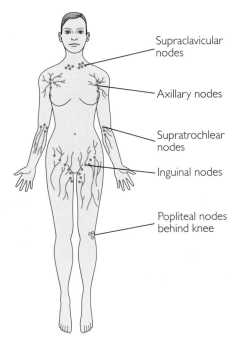

Figure 7.6   Lymphatic nodes of the body

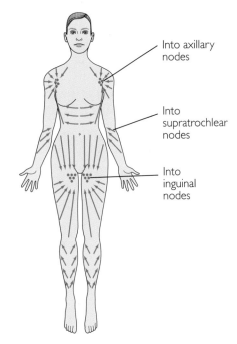

Figure 7.7   Direction of strokes, anterior aspect

Recovery position

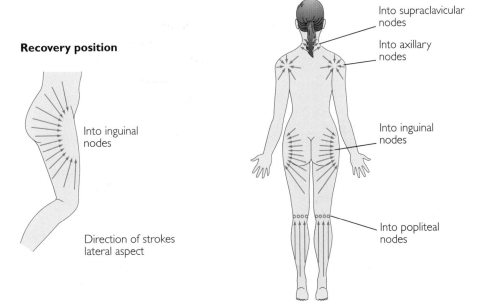

Figure 7.8   Direction of strokes, lateral and posterior aspects

Contraindications

1　Skin diseases and disorders, sunburn.

2　Broken capillaries (thread veins) or varicose veins.

3　Recent stretch marks and scars.

4　Loose, crêpey skin and ageing thin skin.

5　Bruises.

6　Thin bony areas.

7　Very hairy areas.

8　Breast tissue.

9　Thrombosis.

10　Phlebitis.

Figure 7.9　Body vacuum suction with electric current

Dangers

1　Bruising of the area caused by poor technique. Bruising may be caused:

　(a)　If the pressure is too high.

　(b)　By pulling the cup off before releasing the vacuum.

　(c)　By over treating the area with too many strokes or too long a treatment.

　(d)　By pushing the cup downwards instead of lifting and gliding.

2　Making thread veins worse if they are not avoided.

3　Overstretching ageing, thin skin.

Precautions

1　Select the correct size of cup to fit the area (the largest possible without losing suction).

2　Check the pressure on yourself.

3　Apply sufficient oil to the area to facilitate the movement of the cup and provide a seal.

4　Lift enough flesh, but do not exceed 20 per cent of the cup.

5　Lift the cup and move it in a straight line to the nearest set of lymph nodes. (Do not work over the nodes.)

6　Release pressure before lifting the cup off the area.

7　Overlap the previous stroke by 1 cm (½ in) to ensure even coverage.

8　Do not over treat the area.

Treatment technique

Preparation of the client

1　Place the client in a well-supported and comfortable position.

2   Check that all jewellery has been removed.

3   Check for contraindications.

4   Explain the treatment to the client.

5   Select the appropriate pre-heating treatment.

6   If the client has not taken a shower, clean the skin with cologne or surgical spirit.

7   Apply oil or cream to the area to facilitate the movement of the cup and to provide a seal between the cup and the skin.

Procedure

1   Place the machine on a stable base and check the plug, leads and tube.

2   Check the intensity controls are at zero.

3   Collect all commodities.

4   Test the machine. (This may be done by placing a finger over the inlet hole and watching the dial, or by placing the cup on the forearm until suction is felt; this must then be adjusted to suit the flesh on the area being treated.)

5   Select cups of suitable size – the largest possible to fit the area without losing suction.

6   Wipe the cup with disinfectant wipes or surgical spirit swabs.

7   Place the cup on the area and adjust the suction so that the skin fills 20 per cent of the cup. (Break the suction quickly if suction is too high,

otherwise bruising and dilation of capillaries may occur.)

8   Lift the cup and glide it in a straight line towards the nearest set of lymph nodes that drain the area.

Pressing the cup down instead of lifting can be painful and may cause bruising.

9   Break the suction by removing finger from the hole on the cup. If there is no hole, depress the flesh with the little finger under the rim of the cup or use the thumb of the other hand to depress the flesh.

The pressure must be released before the cup is lifted otherwise bruising and dilated capillaries may occur.

10   Move to the adjacent area, overlapping the last stroke by 1 cm or ½ in only. Continue until all the area is covered. Return over the first stroke and cover the area five to ten times depending on the type of flesh and desired effect.

Do not repeat the stroke over the same area without moving on – this can cause dilated capillaries.

The rhythm should be of medium even speed, not too fast or too slow. The sequence should be as follows:

(a)   Place the cup on the body part, filling 20 per cent of the cup.

(b)   Lift the cup and move it in a straight line towards the nearest lymph nodes draining that area.

(c) Release the pressure.

(d) The next stroke should overlap the last stroke by 1 cm or ½ in if possible.

11 At the end of the treatment, effleurage the area and remove oil from the body part.

12 Clean the cups and tube – wash in hot water and detergent, dry and wipe with disinfectant wipes, or soak in disinfectant.

Vacuum suction should form part of a treatment routine – pre-heating followed by gyratory vibrator or manual massage to warm and soften the area and increase circulation. This can be followed by vacuum suction then electrical muscle stimulation (EMS) or exercises.

If galvanic treatment has been given, do not use vacuum suction over the area of the pads as the skin will be very sensitive. Vacuum suction can be done prior to galvanic treatment to decongest the area.

REMEMBER! Feedback and after care.

Pulsating Multi-cup Vacuum Suction

Multi-cup vacuum suction machines are manufactured for treating localized, large areas. They have the advantage of not requiring the constant effort of the therapist. However, care and practice is necessary to select the correct high and low pressure in each individual cup. This treatment is only suitable for obese clients with a considerable covering of adipose tissue.

Machines

These machines are similar to the single cup vacuum suction units, but are larger and have four to six outlets (each outlet has its own shut-off valve). Plastic tubing connects the cups to the outlets. The cups come in various sizes and are selected to suit the area being treated. The reduced pressure created by these machines is always 'pulsed'. This allows for a period of high suction and a period of low suction.

The high suction time must be carefully controlled to produce the required effect, but not so high that it damages capillaries causing bruising of tissues. The low suction period must be just high enough to keep the cup on the part, but it must allow the tissues to relax. Treatments should commence with longer periods of

Figure 7.10 A vacuum suction unit for facial and body treatment constant and pulsating action

low suction. Periods of high suction should be gradually increased according to the client's tolerance.

Treatment technique

Preparation of the client

Prepare the client as for gliding body vacuum suction (see page 132).

Procedure

1 Place the machine on a suitable stable base and check that the plugs and leads are secure.

2 Check that the intensity controls are at zero.

3 Collect all commodities.

4 Test the machine.

5 Commence treatment with a gliding method to introduce the treatment to client.

6 Position the first cup, open its valve, adjust the main control until the required 'lift' of flesh is obtained, switch on the pulse rhythm and adjust the control so that the flesh relaxes, but the cup does not fall off.

7 Repeat this for all the cups.

8 Adjust the pulse to alter the length and degree of 'lift' if necessary.

9 Slide the cups to a new area at regular intervals to prevent over treating and bruising.

10 At the end of the treatment, switch off each valve in turn and remove the cups.

11 Use a gliding single-cup method to drain the area for around 5 minutes at the end of the treatment. Pulsating treatments can be applied for 10–15 minutes depending on the client's skin reaction and tolerance.

12 Wash all the cups and tubes with hot water and detergent, dry and wipe over with disinfectant wipes, or soak them in disinfectant.

REMEMBER! Feedback and after care.

Combined systems

New sophisticated systems are now available which utilize the underlying principles of vacuum suction but combine these with additional techniques.

- The Celluloss concept from Biogenie combines vacuum suction with a simultaneously applied electric current.
- The Endermologie concept from CACI combines vacuum suction with a 'lifting, rolling' massage action.

The highly individual patented heads of these designer-led systems have different and very specific methods of application. The protocol and step by step routines must be adhered to. They require specialist tuition and demonstration from the manufacturers.

The instructions for use must be understood and accurately followed.

The effects produced will be similar to body vacuum suction but enhanced by the effect of the current or the massage.

Figure 7.11 The patented Celluloss head showing the metal contacts which deliver the electrical current, and the central hole for the vacuum suction.

Figure 7.12 One phase of the treatment above

Figure 7.13 The Endermologie system

The treatment is used:

- To soften and aid the dispersal of fat from specific areas providing the client is on a diet.
- To soften areas of cellulite and improve body contours.
- To increase lymphatic drainage thus improving areas of stasis and fluid retention.
- To increase the circulation to, and improve the condition of, the skin.

SUMMARY

- This treatment speeds up the flow of lymph in the lymphatic vessels and therefore removes waste products from the area more quickly and reduces any oedema in the area. It also increases the circulation to the area, bringing oxygen and nutrients to the body part and removing waste products.

- **The lymphatic system** Small blind end tubes, called lymphatic capillaries, form a network through tissue spaces between cells; they join to form larger lymphatic vessels. These vessels drain into lymph nodes where lymph is filtered; lymph nodes also produce lymphocytes. Afferent lymph vessels enter the nodes; efferent lymph vessels leave the nodes. Lymph vessels eventually form lymph trunks which drain into the thoracic duct or into the right lymphatic duct and then into the right and left subclavian veins.

lymph from tissue spaces → lymph capillaries → lymph nodes → lymph trunks → thoracic duct / right lymphatic duct → subclavian veins

The main lymph nodes of the face and body

Facial nodes	Body nodes
Superficial cervical	Axillary nodes (in the armpit or axilla)
Deep cervical	Inguinal nodes (in groin)
Posterior auricular – mastoid	Supratrochlear nodes (at elbow)
Anterior auricular – parotid	Popliteal nodes (behind knee)
Buccal	Supraclavicular nodes (above the clavicle – drain the dowager's hump region)
Submental	
Submandibular	
Occipital	

- Vacuum suction on the face is used for general and deep cleansing and to stimulate and improve the condition of the dry, dehydrated skin.
- The treatment time for general cleansing is 5 minutes.

summary continues overleaf

summary continued from previous page

- The treatment time for deep cleansing is 10–12 minutes.
- The treatment time to improve condition of skin is 10–12 minutes.
- The above timings depend on the skin reaction.
- Vacuum suction is used on the body in conjunction with other treatments to improve the circulation of the blood and lymph, to aid dispersal of fatty deposits for clients on a diet, to improve areas of cellulite, and to reduce oedema.
- The treatment time will depend on the size of the area to be treated – the larger the area the longer the time needed to cover it (five to ten times).
- The main danger is causing bruising of the area. Bruising may be caused if the pressure is too high; by pulling the cup off before releasing the vacuum; by over treating the area with too many strokes; by pushing the cup down instead of lifting and gliding it.
- Other dangers are making thread veins worse and overstretching ageing skin.

Feedback

Examine the area and ask appropriate questions to obtain feedback, this will indicate if the treatment is effective, suitable and the client is happy.

After care

Give advice on immediate after care and any routine to follow before the next treatment.

QUESTIONS

1 Explain why the treatment is called vacuum suction.
2 Briefly explain how lymph is carried from the tissue spaces to the right and left subclavian veins.
3 Give two functions of lymph nodes and list the main nodes of the face and body.
4 What is meant by 'oedema'?
5 Give six contraindications to facial vacuum suction treatment.
6 Explain the benefits of using vacuum suction on the face.
7 What prior treatment might be used to enhance the effect of vacuum suction to the face?
8 Give three reasons for using vacuum suction on the body.
9 How may the vacuum be released at the end of each stroke?
10 What is the purpose of applying oil to the area?

questions continues overleaf

questions continued from previous page

11   List three dangers associated with vacuum suction treatment.
12   How much flesh should be lifted into the cup?
13   How may bruising be caused in the area of application?
14   Explain how the cups and tubes should be dealt with after treatment, to ensure high standards of hygiene.

Oral questions

Facial vacuum suction treatments

1   Why does the flesh rise into the cup?
2   How do you control the degree of suction?
3   How much flesh should be lifted into the cup?
4   Why did you select this treatment for the client?
5   Why did you follow a particular pattern when moving the ventouse over the skin?
6   Name the lymph nodes you were working towards.
7   How did you release the suction at the end of the stroke?
8   Why is it important to release the suction before lifting the ventouse off the part?
9   How do you hold the ventouse?
10   How do you clean the ventouse after treatment?
11   How long is a vacuum suction treatment?
12   What procedure would you follow after the treatment?

Body vacuum suction treatments

1   What are the methods of applying vacuum suction to the body?
2   When would you select vacuum suction as a suitable treatment?
3   (a) Can any harm come to the client when having vacuum suction?
     (b) How can you avoid these problems?
4   How would you ensure good, even coverage?
5   How would you select the cup size?
6   How would you decide when to stop the treatment?
7   How would vacuum suction be combined with other treatments?
8   Would you use vacuum suction after galvanic treatment?

8 Galvanic Treatment

OBJECTIVES

After you have studied this chapter you will be able to:

1 Identify a galvanic unit, its terminals and electrodes.

2 List the treatments which use the galvanic current.

3 Describe the type of current used in galvanic treatments.

4 Briefly explain the chemical electrolysis of sodium chloride solution (salt or saline solution).

5 Briefly describe the effects of galvanic treatment to the body using the pads soaked in salt solution.

6 Explain the uses of disincrustation treatment.

7 Carry out disincrustation treatment, paying due consideration to maximum efficiency, comfort, safety and hygiene.

8 Explain the uses of iontophoresis treatment.

9 Carry out iontophoresis treatment, paying due consideration to maximum efficiency, comfort, safety and hygiene.

10 Explain the uses of body galvanism.

11 Explain the dangers of galvanic application to the body.

12 List the precautions to be taken during galvanic application to the body.

13 Treat the client with body galvanism, paying due consideration to maximum efficiency, comfort, safety and hygiene.

Galvanic treatments use a direct current. It flows in one direction and has polarity.

Figure 8.1 is a photograph of a galvanic machine or unit. This is one of the larger models and may be used for both facial and body work. Galvanic treatments use a low voltage direct (constant) current, sometimes called a galvanic current. This current flows in one direction only and has polarity. One electrode is negatively charged (called the **cathode**), while the other is positively charged (called the **anode**). Galvanic treatments may be used on the face or body and

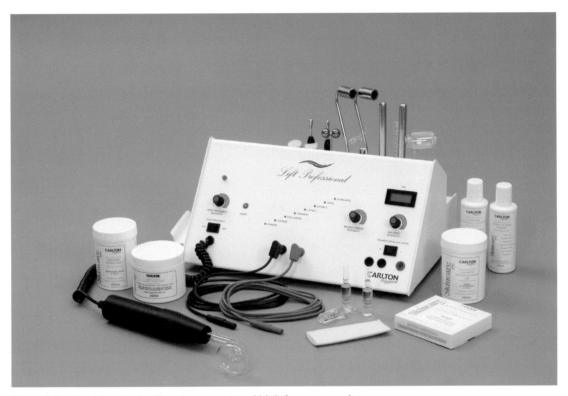

Figure 8.1   Combined galvanic, microcurrent and high frequency unit

are given specific names:

Facial treatments

1 **Disincrustation** This is a deep cleansing treatment; the effects at the cathode are used to remove the build up of sebum and keratinized cells and to soften the skin of the face.

2 **Iontophoresis** or **ion repulsion** This treatment uses specially manufactured products which are repelled into the skin by appropriate electrodes. It is suitable for many skin types as a variety of products are available to suit different skin conditions.

Body treatments

1 **Iontophoresis** Specially manufactured anti-cellulite products are used to soften and aid the dispersal of hard fat (cellulite).

2 **Body galvanism** This treatment uses the softening effect under the cathode when using a sodium chloride (salt) solution under the electrode, to treat areas of cellulite.

The effects produced by these treatments are dependent on:

1 The chemistry of electrolysis.
2 The laws of physics which state that like charges repel and opposite charges attract.

The first part of this chapter explains these principles, and it is recommended that you study and understand them before commencing treatments. This knowledge will enable you to select the most appropriate and effective treatment to suit the needs of the client. It will also enable you to fully explain the treatment to the client.

Underpinning knowledge

Read the sections on elements, compounds, atoms, ions and electrolysis in Chapter 4.

Electrolysis of Sodium Chloride Solution

An electrolyte is a chemical compound which conducts a current.

A solution containing salt and water is an electrolyte. In solution, the sodium chloride will ionize and the water will ionize slightly.

Sodium chloride will ionize giving sodium (+) ions and chloride (−) ions

$$NaCl \rightarrow Na^+ \text{ and } Cl^-$$

Water will ionize giving hydrogen (+) ions and hydroxyl (−) ions

$$H_2O \rightarrow H^+ \text{ and } OH^-$$

These ions move freely in the solution; when a direct current is applied to the solution by means of two electrodes, the current will flow through the electrolyte. The electrodes will be charged depending on their connections to the battery or machine. One will be negatively charged, the cathode. The other will be positively charged, the anode. When the current is

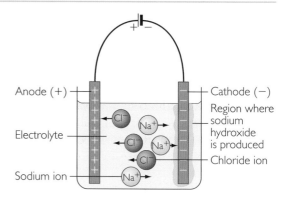

Figure 8.2   Electrolysis of sodium chloride solution

switched on, the ions will move away from or towards the electrodes. This occurs because:

1 Like charges repel.
2 Opposite charges attract.

Therefore, the cations (+) will move towards the cathode (−) and the anions (−) will move towards the anode (+).

When the ions reach the electrode with the opposite charge, some are discharged and certain chemical reactions take place.

The following reactions are used in galvanic treatments:

- At the cathode (−) the sodium ion (Na^+) reacts with the hydroxyl ion (OH^-) in the water producing the alkali sodium hydroxide (NaOH) and hydrogen (H_2) gas.
- At the anode (+) the chloride ion (Cl^-) reacts with the hydrogen ions (H^+) in the water producing hydrochloric acid (HCl) and oxygen (O_2) gas.

The formation of the alkali sodium hydroxide at the cathode is used in facial disincrustation and body galvanism. A current applied to the body by means of two electrodes will be carried through the tissues. This happens because tissue fluid contains a high percentage of salts and is an electrolyte. A pad of lint or foam soaked in salt solution and placed under the cathode and moved over or strapped to the skin will result in the production of sodium hydroxide under the pad. This has a softening effect on the tissues. At the same time, hydrochloric acid will be produced under the anode. This hardens the tissues.

The Effects of Direct Current Application

The following text explains why specific treatments are effective. Therapists who do not require such details should proceed to the sections on specific treatments where the appropriate effects are listed.

When a direct current is applied to the body certain effects are produced at the electrodes also known as 'poles'. These effects are known as 'polar effects'. Other effects are produced in the tissues between the electrodes or poles; these are known as 'interpolar effects'.

Polar effects

These occur immediately beneath the electrodes.

Alkaline reactions at the cathode

The production of the strong alkali, sodium hydroxide, at the cathode (−) is very irritating to the skin, and great care must be taken to avoid chemical burns to the skin (see page 171 regarding technique). The alkali saponifies the sebum and has a drying effect on the skin. It breaks down the keratin in keratinized cells, thus softening the skin and scar tissue. It neutralizes the acidity of the skin, destroying the acid mantle, therefore, reducing its germicidal properties.

Acid reactions at the anode

The production of hydrochloric acid at the anode (+) also has an irritating effect, but is less marked than at the cathode. It can, however, cause burns to the skin, but these will differ in appearance from burns produced under the cathode.

The tissues under the anode tend to tighten, harden and improve in condition – this is due to the hardening effect of the acid and also to the release of oxygen which will nourish and improve the vitality of the cells. The production of acid increases the acidic protection of the skin and increases its germicidal properties.

Vasodilation at both electrodes

> Vasodilation occurs under both electrodes but is more marked under the cathode due to greater irritation.

The irritating nature of the alkali and acid at the poles produces vasodilation under both electrodes. It is more marked and lasts longer under the cathode due to greater irritation. Vasodilation occurs because skin reacts to irritation by a process known as the 'triple response'.

Firstly, irritation of the cells causes release of histamine – this results in dilation of the capillaries, producing erythema or reddening of the skin.

Secondly, further reddening is produced by 'axon reflex', which produces dilation of arterioles in the area. Nerve impulses travelling from pain receptors through the axon can travel directly through another axon branch to the arteriol wall without proceeding to the central nervous system. These impulses stimulate the muscle wall of the arteriol to relax and the vessel to dilate.

Thirdly, more severe irritation will result in increased permeability of capillary walls and plasma will pass out into the tissues. This will increase the amount of tissue fluid in the area. It can be seen that the irritation under the electrodes will produce vasodilation giving hyperaemia, erythema and heat.

These effects are far greater under the cathode ($-$) due to the intense irritating quality of sodium hydroxide and the release of active hydrogen.

Production of heat under both electrodes

An increase in blood flow to an area will raise the temperature of the area. During galvanic treatments, the degree of heat

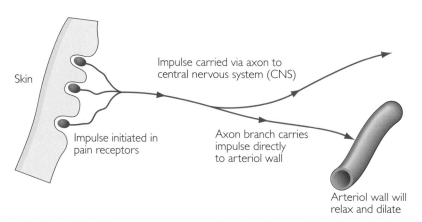

Skin

Impulse carried via axon to central nervous system (CNS)

Impulse initiated in pain receptors

Axon branch carries impulse directly to arteriol wall

Arteriol wall will relax and dilate

Figure 8.3   Impulses transmitted from sensory receptor directly to the arteriol wall resulting in dilation produced will be directly proportional to the intensity of the current, the time for which it flows and the resistance offered to the current. Again the heating under the cathode (−) is greater than under the anode (+) due to greater vasodilation.

Particular attention must be paid to technique when applying galvanic treatments in order to minimize any risk of causing thermal burns, (see page 163).

Excitability of nerves under both electrodes

- The cathode (−) reduces the resting potential difference (PD) of a nerve, thus increasing conductivity and excitability.

- The anode (+) increases the resting PD of the nerve thus reducing conductivity and excitability. Prolonged treatment may result in numbing of the area – an analgesic effect at the anode.

Fluid content

At the cathode there is an increase in tissue fluid. This is partly due to the increased permeability of vessel walls and also because water molecules move away from the anode (+) towards the cathode (−). This effect can be used to soften scars.

At the anode there is a decrease in tissue fluid which results in hardening of the tissues.

Ion repulsion

The effects of repelling ions into the skin (iontophoresis) will be specific to the type of manufactured product selected.

Many products are produced in different forms (e.g. gels, ampules and serums) for the treatment of various conditions. The manufacturer's instructions must be carefully read and adhered to and the correct electrode must be selected to repel the ions in the gel. Like charges repel, therefore:

- If the gel contains negatively charged beneficial ions, the cathode (−) must be used as the active electrode.

- If the gel contains positively charged beneficial ions, then the anode (+) is used as the active electrode.

- The inactive electrode is placed elsewhere on the body to complete the circuit.

Interpolar effects

In addition to the effects immediately under the poles, there are effects in the tissues between the electrodes.

Blood circulation

There is an increase in blood circulating through the tissues. Therefore, nutrients and oxygen are brought to the area and metabolites are removed more quickly.

Lymphatic circulation

There is an increase in lymphatic circulation, thus removing waste products more quickly.

Increased cell metabolism

There is an increase in the permeability of cell walls resulting in increased cell metabolism. Chemical compounds within the cells are split into ions making them easier to remove.

Reduction in blood pressure

Body galvanic treatments reduce both diastolic and systolic pressure. This should be borne in mind if clients suffer from low blood pressure.

Physiological effects at the cathode

1 Strong alkali sodium hydroxide is formed which is very irritating to the tissues, it:

    (a) Saponifies sebum.

    (b) Breaks down keratin.

    (c) Reduces the acidity of the skin.

    (d) Destroys the acid mantle reducing the skin's protective function against micro-organisms.

    (e) Has a drying effect on the skin.

2 Marked vasodilation with hyper-aemia and erythema (due to heat and irritation).

3 Heat is produced; the degree of heat depends on the intensity of the current, the time for which it flows and the resistance to the current.

4 Increased excitability and conductivity of nerves.

5 Increased tissue fluid drawn to the area (this effect can be used to soften scars).

Physiological effects at the anode

1 Hydrochloric acid is formed which is irritating to the tissues and:

    (a) Increases the acidity of the skin.

    (b) Improves and restores the acid mantle and the skin's protective function.

    (c) Tightens and hardens the tissues.

2 Less marked vasodilation, hyper-aemia and erythema (due to less heat and irritation).

3 Mild heat produced.

4 Oxygen is released improving the condition of the tissues.

5 Decreased excitability and conductivity of nerves, prolonged treatment can produce numbing of the area (analgesic effect).

Physiological effects in the tissues between the electrodes (interpolar)

1 Increased blood flow through the area.

2 Increased lymphatic flow through the area.

3 Increased permeability of blood vessel walls.

4 Improved cell metabolism.

5 Slight reduction in blood pressure.

Galvanic Units and Systems

There is a wide variety of machines on the market for use as facial units, body units and combined facial and body units. Low voltage direct current is produced by a battery or modified AC mains. This current is applied to the body using electrodes connected to the machine by leads. One electrode will be negative, called the cathode. The other will be positive, called the anode. All machines have intensity controls and a milliammeter to indicate current flow. Machines may have single sockets for each pair of leads (i.e. each connecting jack will divide into two leads) or the machine may have independent sockets for each lead. In this instance, the connectors on the machine are usually coloured red or black.

If the unit has independent colour sockets for each lead (often used in facial systems), the red and black connecting leads must be plugged into matching coloured sockets. Units with single sockets have a red or black pin to identify polarity.

Both facial and body systems usually include a polarity reversal switch. This is intended to reverse the polarity should the therapist require to do so during the treatment. Because machines are not standardized, the polarity switch may be misinterpreted by the therapist and this can lead to incorrect treatment. It is vital to refer to each individual manufacturer's instruction manual to ensure understanding and correct use of machine.

> Ensure that you understand how each galvanic unit works. Read the manufacturer's instruction for each unit.

Examples of wording and switching found on different units

On the unit below, the polarity indicator uses two types of instructions: symbols ('+' and '−') and wording ('normal' and 'reverse'). Manufacturers will consider the wording 'normal' and 'reverse' to automatically indicate the *normal* law of colour coding (i.e. red = positive and black = negative).

When the switch is moved to positive, the red lead is positive (+). When switched to negative the red lead is negative (−).

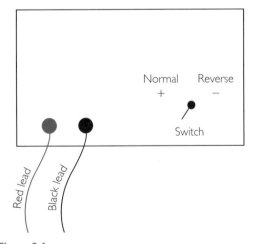

Figure 8.4

Some manufacturers help to make the polarity switch more visually obvious. The ISIS module galvanic has independent connecting plugs as in Figure 8.5 and the red and black leads plug in as normal.

Figure 8.5

Figure 8.6

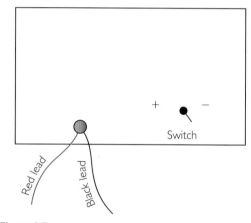

Figure 8.7

When the switch is moved to the left, the normal position, a red light illuminates the red connector indicating that this connector is positive. When the switch is moved to the right (i.e. reverse), a red light illuminates the black connector indicating that this has now become the positive connector.

The greatest confusion arises when using a single socket outlet. The two leads may be coloured (one red and one black) or may be buff coloured with the terminal ends coloured (one red, one black).

If the polarity switch uses only symbols as above, it is essential to read the manufacturer's instructions to establish how the system has been designed as the switch could be wired in two different ways.

1 On some machines, the design may be such that when the switch is set to the '+' symbol, the red terminal is the positive (+) and the black terminal is the negative (−). When the switch is set to the '−' symbol, the red becomes negative (−) and the black becomes positive (+). This is fairly straightforward as the red lead is thought of as the master lead. *But:*

2 On other machines, when the switch is flicked towards the '−', then the black lead is negative (−) and the red lead is positive (+). By reversing the switch the black lead has become positive (+) and the red lead negative (−).

NOTE! This can lead to a great deal of confusion; therefore, always check with the manufacturer's instructions.

It is always vital to check the polarity output of each machine oneself. This can be done in different ways:

1 To check the polarity, hold both electrodes in your hand and increase the intensity: the negative electrode/pole will always be the more irritating. This test is the easiest to perform, but is not as definite as the water test.

2 Hold the leads in a beaker of water and increase the intensity: bubbles of hydrogen will be seen at the cathode ($-$).

3 Red litmus paper could also be used – this will turn blue under the cathode.

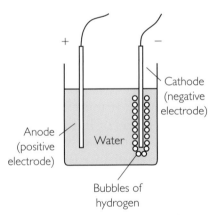

Figure 8.8 Hydrogen bubbles at the cathode

Therapists must always ensure that they understand all the components

of the machines in order to give effective treatments. Older machines are still found in some departments and salons. These will differ in design and may have a 'shunt' switch. This switch, when moved from 0 to 10, will multiply the current by 10. Therefore, on the meter:

- a reading of 1 mA (milliamp) indicates an output of 10 mA

- a reading of 2 mA indicates an output of 20 mA.

These current intensities are far too high and great care must be taken if using these machines.

The terminology applied to the electrodes is also confusing. One electrode will always be negatively charged, called the cathode. The other will be positively charged, called the anode. Normal colour coding indicates that the cathode is black and the anode is red, but as previously explained, this may not always apply.

Various names are also used when describing the electrode which is producing the required effect and the one merely completing the circuit:

Active – Passive   Active – Indifferent
Active – Inactive   Differential – Passive

Facial Galvanic Treatments

The direct or galvanic current is used in two ways on the face to improve cleanliness, tone texture and condition of the skin. The methods are known as **disincrustation** and **iontophoresis**.

Facial Disincrustation Treatments

Disincrustation treatment is based on the chemistry of electrolysis and uses the chemical reaction produced when a direct current is passed through saline solution, or a specific product.

The treatment requires a source of direct current applied to the body via two electrodes: a cathode (−) which must be the active electrode and an anode (+) which is the inactive electrode. It also requires a salt solution as an electrolyte (made by mixing 2 teaspoonfuls of salt to 1 litre of water). There are manufactured products available which produce the same effect but will be more costly.

The alkali, sodium hydroxide, formed under the cathode (−) will soften the build up of sebum, break down keratinized cells of the superficial layer of the skin, open pores and release blockages. It is therefore used as a general and deep cleansing treatment.

Electrodes

The anode (+) is the inactive electrode and must be placed in a comfortable position on the client to complete the circuit. It may be a metal rod, which is held in the client's hand, or a metal plate, which is placed on the upper arm. In both cases, it must be covered with moist lint or dense foam which must be of even texture 1 cm or ½ inch thick and larger by 1 cm or ½ inch than the electrode.

The cathode (−) is the active electrode and is the one used on the face for disincrustation treatments. There are several varieties:

1 Disc electrode – this is the one generally used. It must be covered by several layers of lint moistened with saline solution or specially manufactured disincrustation products.

2 Tweezer electrode.

Uses at the cathode (−)

1 General cleansing of a combination and greasy skin.

2 Deep cleansing of a seborrhoeic skin.

3 Stimulation of a sluggish skin with build up of keratinized cells and comedomes.

A careful skin analysis must be carried out before treatment to ensure that the skin type is suitable for disincrustation.

Figure 8.9   A facial galvanic unit with electrodes

Although fluid is temporarily drawn to the cathode (−), this treatment should not be used on a mature or dry/dehydrated skin as the caustic effect of the alkali, sodium hydroxide, would exacerbate the condition.

> Disincrustation treatment is not suitable for a mature or dry/dehydrated skin.

Effects at the cathode (−)

1 The alkali, sodium hydroxide, formed will saponify sebum and soften the skin; the pores relax releasing the sebum. It will also break down the keratin in the superficial layers of the skin, thus softening and cleansing the area.

2 Fluid drawn towards the cathode (−) will soften the skin. This hydrating effect is only temporary.

3 It causes vasodilation with hyperaemia and erythema; the increase in circulation brings nutrients and oxygen to nourish the skin and removes waste products. This will improve the condition of the skin and improve the colour of sallow, sluggish skin.

4 It increases cell metabolism, which improves the condition of the skin.

5 The alkali, sodium hydroxide, alters the pH of the skin, destroying the acid mantle. This is an undesirable effect and is corrected by reversing the polarity at the end of the treatment for 2–4 minutes.

Uses at the anode (+) when the polarity is reversed

The effects at the anode (+) can be used to improve the tone and texture of the skin and refine a skin with large, open pores. The hydrochloric acid formed will tighten the tissue and help to close the pores. It will restore the acid mantle and improve the skin's resistance to infection. The oxygen will help to nourish and revitalize the tissues.

Effects at the anode (+) when the polarity is reversed

1 The formation of hydrochloric acid restores the acid mantle.

2 The acid tightens and firms the skin.

3 Tissue fluid moves away from the anode.

4 There is little vasodilation with erythema.

5 The release of oxygen revitalizes the tissues.

Contraindications

1 Lack of skin sensitivity, which may be caused by damage to or pressure on nerves, neurological disorders, scarring. Bell's palsy or dental treatments, etc. Always check with hot and cold and with blunt and sharp tests (see page 154).

2 Cuts and abrasions (cover small cuts with petroleum jelly and plaster).

3 Metal pins or plates around the head or excessive fillings.

4 Hypersensitive skins (e.g. rosacea, dermatitis and telangiectasis).

5   Pustular acne with inflamed areas.

6   Highly nervous clients.

Dangers

1   **Burns.** The danger of burns with facial galvanic treatment correctly applied is minimal as the time of application is short, current intensity low and the electrode is moving continually.

2   **Shock.** There is danger of shock if the current is turned up or down suddenly, if the electrodes are lifted off the skin during treatment or if the resistance of the skin drops suddenly.

Precautions

1   Check for contraindications.

2   Test for skin sensitivity.

3   Check that all jewellery has been removed.

4   Check the machine and test it on yourself.

5   Ensure that salt crystals have completely dissolved.

6   Saturate the gauze or pad evenly.

7   Place the active electrode on a sensitive area, such as the forehead, and turn the current up very slowly.

8   Keep the pad moist during treatment (use a dropper if necessary).

9   Turn the current down slowly before lifting the electrode.

10 Speak to the client throughout the treatment.

> Keep the electrode on the forehead, switch on and turn up very slowly.

Treatment technique

Preparation of the client

1   Place the client in a well-supported and comfortable position.

2   Check that all jewellery has been removed.

3   Check for contraindications.

4   Explain the treatment to the client.

5   Cleanse and tone the skin.

6   Check for sensitivity to hot and cold. Use two test tubes: one containing hot water and one containing cold water. Tell the client to close her eyes. Touch randomly over the face with the hot and cold test tubes, asking the client to identify which one is touching her. Also test her sensitivity to blunt and sharp using an orange stick/blunt needle and cotton wool (proceed as for hot and cold test). If the client is able to identify both hot/cold and blunt/sharp, her sensation is intact and the treatment may proceed. If she is repeatedly unable to identify either, her sensation is defective and treatment should not be carried out.

7   Apply a little petroleum jelly around the eye to prevent 'flash'. (This is an uncomfortable feeling which may happen if the electrode moves too near the eye.)

Procedure

1 Position the machine on a stable base and check that the plugs, leads and terminals are secure and away from water.

2 Check that the intensity control is at zero.

3 Collect all commodities.

4 Test the machine: hold both electrodes in one hand and increase the intensity of the current.

5 Prepare a saline solution – stir 2 teaspoonfuls of salt into 1 litre of water; make sure that all the crystals have dissolved. (Or select disincrustation gel if this is to be used.)

6 Select the appropriate electrodes and plug them into the machine.

7 Saturate all lint or sponges in saline solution: if you are using a gauze mask, saturate this; if you are using a manufacturer's gel, apply this thinly and evenly over greasy areas of the face, or use it to saturate the gauze.

8 Place a dampened cover around the inactive electrode (anode (+)) and give it to the client to hold if it is a rod electrode, or strap it on to the upper arm if it is a plate electrode.

9 Secure the saturated gauze/lint to the active electrode (the cathode (−)).

10 Explain the sensation to the client and ask her to report any discomfort.

11 Place the cathode on the client's skin. Choose an area of high sensitivity (e.g. the forehead), and switch on.

12 Turn the current up slowly, moving the electrode on the face. Very low current is needed, up to a maximum of 2 mA. This must be within the client's tolerance.

13 As soon as the client feels a prickling sensation, turn the current down slightly.

Turn the intensity up and down very slowly.

14 Move the electrode slowly over face and neck using a circular movement. Cover the face or greasy areas evenly for up to 10 minutes or according to manufacturer's instructions.

15 At the end of the treatment turn the intensity down very slowly and switch off with electrode still in contact with the face.

16 Replace the lint or gauze and reverse the polarity of the machine.

17 Place the electrode on the face again and repeat the procedure for 2–5 minutes. (This will restore the pH of the skin.)

18 Turn the intensity down slowly as before and switch off.

19 The face must be thoroughly wiped over with damp cotton wool. Then apply toner and blot with tissue.

20 Clean the electrodes – wash them with hot water and detergent and wipe over with a disinfectant wipe.

Make-up should not be worn for 8 hours.

Keep the electrode in contact with the skin throughout the treatment.

REMEMBER! Feedback and after care.

Facial Iontophoresis Treatment

This uses a direct current to introduce beneficial products into the skin. The treatment is based on the principle that like charges repel and opposite charges attract.

A source of direct current is applied to the face or body and the electrodes are used to repel ions of beneficial substances into the skin.

Manufacturers produce a wide range of gels/serums, etc., suitable for various skin conditions. The products contain ions which carry either negative or positive charges. The success of this treatment is dependent upon:

1 Correct identification of the skin condition.

2 The selection of the appropriate product for the skin condition.

3 The selection of the appropriate electrode to repel the product. If the product is negatively charged, the cathode (−) will be the active electrode. The cathode (−) will repel the anions (−) in the product into the skin. If the product is positively charged, the anode (+) will be the active electrode. The anode (+) will repel the cations (+) in the product into the skin.

This movement of anions is called *anaphoresis* and the movement of cations is called *cataphoresis*.

Electrodes

Types of electrode:

1 Ball electrode.

2 Roller electrode.

Gels and serums that are repelled under electrodes are thought to achieve deeper penetration than manual applications. Penetration is thought to be less than 1 mm, but deeper absorption may be achieved via the capillary circulation and transport through cell membranes.

Research has indicated that low level intensity currents and low ionic concentrations may well be as effective as high intensity currents and high ionic concentrations (on the basis that a few ions entering slowly will find it easier to enter the skin than a mass of ions all with the same charge repelling each other as they are forced through). However, some products may require certain intensities for their repulsion, and manufacturers sometimes offer guidelines which should be carefully followed. When products with-out guidelines are used, it should be borne in mind that a low current is often effective.

> Accurate skin analysis and selection of the appropriate product is essential to the success of the treatment.

Uses

This form of treatment can be used for a wide variety of skin conditions. A careful skin analysis must be made to diagnose the problem areas. The appropriate prod-uct can then be selected to suit the needs of the client:

1 **Hydration** and **moisturising** Many products are manufactured for moisturising and hydrating a dry and mature skin; serums containing collagen, elastin and placental extracts are particularly beneficial.

2 **Regeneration** Products are available for the repair and regeneration of mature skin and of damaged skin, particularly after exposure to the sun and wind.

3 **Stimulating** Products for stimulating a sluggish, sallow complexion include extracts of seaweed and other marine products. Care must be taken not to over treat with these products.

4 **Improvement of sensitive skins** Gels and serums are available for the treatment of the sensitive couperose skin. Care must be taken when treating these skin types as many conditions

can be exacerbated by the direct current. Rosacea, dermatitis and highly vascular conditions would be contraindicated and should not be treated with galvanic current.

Effects

1 When using iontophoresis the main effect will depend on, and be specific to, the product used. Manufacturers recommend their products for specific skin types and also indicate which electrode should be used for repelling the ions into the skin. The products come in many forms (e.g. gels, ampules, serums, impregnated gauze, etc.) and contain extracts of beneficial substances such as collagen, elastin, placental or herbal extracts of ivy, seaweed, etc. Therefore careful skin analysis must be carried out and the appropriate product selected to achieve the most beneficial outcome for the client. Other effects will be due to stimulation by the direct current.

2 Vasodilation, with hyperaemia and erythema, will increase the circula-tion to the face bringing oxygen and nutrients to improve the condition of the skin.

3 The increase in cell metabolism will improve the condition of the skin.

4 Desquamation is aided due to increased mitotic activity of the basal layer.

5 Improvement in the colour and texture of the skin due to an increase in blood flow and an increase in desquamation.

Contraindications

1   Lack of skin sensitivity.

2   Cuts and abrasions.

3   Metal pins or plates.

4   Hypersensitive skins (e.g. rosacea, dermatitis and telangiectasis).

5   Pustular acne with inflamed areas.

6   Highly nervous clients.

Dangers

1   **Burns** The danger of burns is minimal as the rollers are continually moving and the current intensity is low.

2   **Shock** There is a danger of shock if the current is turned up or down suddenly, or if the intensity is turned up before the electrode is in contact with the face.

Precautions

1   Test the client's skin sensitivity with hot/cold, blunt/sharp.

2   Check that the controls are at zero.

3   Test the current on yourself.

4   Apply the gel or ampule content evenly and thinly over the face. If using a gauze mask, saturate it evenly and make sure that it is applied smoothly to the face with no wrinkling or puckering.

5   Place the rollers on a sensitive area of skin (e.g. the forehead or jaw line) and keep them moving while turning the current up slowly and steadily.

6   Turn the intensity down slightly when the client feels a tingling sensation. (Remember this treatment is more effective with a low intensity current and low ionic concentrations. Turn the current up only within the tolerance of the client.)

7   Move the rollers slowly over the face without breaking contact with the skin.

8   Do not knock the rollers together during treatment as the current will flow from one to the other.

9   Turn the current down slowly before removing the electrodes.

10 Do not allow the skin to become dry during treatment as the treatment would become ineffective.

11 Use petroleum jelly around the eyes. This acts as insulation to prevent 'flash'.

12 Always follow the manufacturer's instructions for the timing of the treatment.

13 Speak to the client throughout the treatment.

Treatment technique

Preparation of the client

1   Place the client in a well-supported and comfortable position.

2   Check that all jewellery has been removed.

3   Check for contraindications.

4   Explain the treatment to the client.

5   Cleanse and tone the skin.

6 Check for skin sensitivity with hot and cold test tubes and an orange stick and cotton wool (see page 154).

7 Apply petroleum jelly around the eye to prevent flash (see page 154).

8 Select the appropriate gel, serum, etc., to suit the skin type and check its charge (i.e. negative or positive).

Procedure

1 Position the machine on a stable base and check that the plugs, leads and terminals are secure.

2 Check that the intensity control is at zero.

3 Select the active roller electrodes and plug them into the machine: negative if the gel is negatively charged; positive if the gel is positively charged.

4 Plug in the inactive electrode into the other socket.

5 Test the machine by holding the active and inactive electrodes in one hand and increasing the intensity of the current.

6 Cover the inactive electrode with moistened foam or lint 1 cm or ½ inch thick and give it to the client to hold, or strap it on to upper arm if it is a plate electrode.

7 Apply gel or the contents of the ampule thinly and evenly over the face and neck, or place saturated gauze over the face and neck.

8 Check that the controls are at zero.

9 Place one roller on to the client's skin, switch on the machine and turn up the current slowly until a tingling sensation is felt, then place the other roller on the other side.

10 Move the rollers over the face without breaking contact with the skin and making sure the rollers do not touch each other. Maintain an even pressure and a slow, rhythmical movement.

11 Ask the client to report any discomfort.

12 Remove one roller and turn the current down slowly and switch off the current before removing the other roller.

13 If necessary, apply a little more gel and use a single ball or fork electrode for concentrated work.

14 Remove excess gel; tone and moisturize. Do not apply make-up for 8 hours.

15 Clean the electrodes – wash them with hot water and detergent, dry and wipe them with a disinfectant wipe.

It is the tolerance of the client which dictates the maximum current from 0.05 mA–2 mA.

High frequency and facial galvanic treatments may be combined to offer effective facial routines.

REMEMBER! Feedback and after care.

Body Galvanic Treatments

The application of a direct current to the tissues of the body will produce certain physiological effects (see page 148). These effects are thought to soften areas of fat or cellulite and aid its dispersal. There are various ways in which the galvanic current is used to produce these effects.

1   **Body galvanism using saline solution** The traditional method of applying the direct current uses electrodes covered with pads soaked in saline solution. This method uses the polar and interpolar effect and is generally called body galvanism. The most irritating and stimulating effects produced at the cathode (−) are used in this method. Therefore the cathode (−) is always the active electrode and is placed over the areas of cellulite while the anode (+) is always placed opposite it or in parallel with it as the inactive electrode.

2   **Iontophoresis galvanic treatment using products** The more modern method uses anti-cellulite gels and ampules containing liquid serum preparations specially manufactured to treat cellulite. These preparations contain charged ions of beneficial substances which are repelled into the skin by use of the appropriate electrode. The gel usually carries negatively charged beneficial ions, therefore the cathode (−) is used to repel them into the tissues. However, if it

carries a positive charge, the anode (+) must be used; always check with the manufacturer's instructions. This method uses the effects of the gel as well as some of the polar and the interpolar effects of the current. This form of treatment is known as body iontophoresis.

3   **Combined systems using body wraps, clays, etc.** Certain modern systems utilize the galvanic current in the treatment of the whole body, via body wraps, clay, etc. These treatments use specially formulated products to achieve the desired results. The current is used for its effect in stimulating the circulation, increasing lymphatic drainage and for stimulating metabolic rate, thus enhancing the effect of the products. These treatments use far lower current intensities than the previous methods, and manufacturer's instructions must be strictly adhered to.

Uses

1   To soften areas of fat/cellulite and aid its absorption.

2   To stimulate the circulation of blood and lymph, thus improving the condition of the skin and tissues.

3   To improve areas of stasis.

4   Body galvanism can be used to soften areas of old, hard scar tissue. The cathode must be used for this as fluid is attracted to the cathode.

Figure 8.10   A body galvanic unit showing body electrodes, pads and strapping

Summary of effects

Polar effects under the cathode (−) (active electrode):

1 When saline solution is used the alkali, sodium hydroxide, is formed. This softens the skin and tissues.

2 Hydrogen is released which is stimulating to the tissues.

3 Vasodilation with hyperaemia and erythema: more blood will flow to the area bringing nutrients and oxygen and removing metabolites.

4 Irritation of sensory nerve endings: it increases the conductivity of nerves.

5 An increase in the water and tissue fluid in the area of the electrode due to increased permeability of vessel walls and to the movement of water molecules away from the anode (+) towards the cathode (−). This will soften the area.

6 Heat is produced under the electrode; the client should feel an even, comfortable warmth.

7 Products, such as gels and ampules, containing negatively charged ions will be repelled into the skin by the cathode (−). The effect produced will be specific to that product (e.g. anti-cellulite products will aid break-down and dispersal of cellulite) and include effects 3–6.

Polar effects under the anode (+)

The anode is usually the inactive electrode in body galvanism. Its effects are not util-ized in the treatment:

1 When saline solution is used hydro-chloric acid is formed, which tightens and hardens the skin and tissues.

2 Oxygen is released which increases the vitality of the tissues.

3 Vasodilation with hyperaemia and erythema result, but this is not as great as under the cathode (−).

4 It decreases the conductivity of nerves and may have an analgesic effect under the pad.

5 A decrease in water content as water molecules move away from the anode (+) towards the cathode (−).

6 Heat is produced under the electrode.

7 Products containing positively charged ions will be repelled into the skin by the anode (+) and effects 2–7 will apply.

Interpolar effects

1 An increase in circulation.

2 An increase in metabolic rate.

3 An increase in lymphatic drainage.

4 The lowering of blood pressure.

Contraindications

1 Lack of skin sensitivity may be due to neurological disorders, injury, scar tissue, etc.

2 Cuts or abrasions; small cuts can be covered with petroleum jelly and waterproof plaster.

3 Extensive scar tissue.

4 Other skin conditions, such as eczema and psoriasis.

5 Metal pins or plates in the area to be treated.

6 Treatment around the abdomen must not be carried out on anyone with an IUD coil.

7 Low blood pressure.

8 Pregnancy.

9 Any medication in the form of ointments that have been applied to the skin, such as Algipan, as these will sensitize the area. (Always wash skin thoroughly to avoid this possibility.)

Dangers

The great danger with the application of direct current to the body is the produc-tion of burns, both chemical and, to a lesser extent, thermal. Burns are caused by poor technique of application and *must* be avoided. An awareness of the nature and causes of galvanic burns will enable the therapist to develop good technique, thus ensuring that burns do not occur.

Thermal burns – caused by a build up of heat

An increase in blood flow to an area will result in the production of heat to that area. The amount of heat produced will be directly proportional to the intensity, time and resistance. Because the processes of conduction, convection and radiation are restricted under the pads, there is a build up of heat.

Causes of thermal burns

If the intensity of the current is high, the time during which it flows is too long or if the resistance to the current is high, there is a danger of producing a thermal burn. The intensity and time of current flow must be carefully controlled and careful consideration must be given to avoid areas of high resistance. Care must be taken to avoid large freckles and areas of hard tissue, such as scars. If scars are being treated, the current intensity must be kept very low, below 2 mA.

The most common causes of high resistance burns are:

(a) pads being unevenly saturated, giving rise to dry/moist spots resulting in high areas of resistance (dry) and low areas of resistance (moist);

(b) unevenness within the pads preventing good, even skin contact;

(c) gaps and air spaces allowed between the skin and the electrode. This happens if a stiff electrode does not adapt to the rounded contour of the body.

Burns may also occur if the client is lying with full body weight on the electrode. This pressure limits the circulating blood and its action of conducting heat away from the area. Therefore, if the posterior aspect of the body is being treated, clients should lie in the prone position (face down) and vice versa.

Tight rubber bandages also produce ischaemia (lack of blood flow); they should apply even firm pressure over the electrode but not be so tight as to occlude the circulation.

Chemical burns caused by a build up of chemicals

There is a greater risk of chemical burns than heat burns, and the risk is greater under the cathode (−) than under the anode (+) because the strong alkali, sodium hydroxide, causes destruction and softening of the tissues. A red sore mark appears immediately, and this later changes to a grey oozing wound. These wounds take a long time to heal and should be treated with care. Cover with a dry, sterile dressing, taking care that the wound does not become infected.

Burns under the anode (+) are more rare due to the low concentration of hydrochloric acid. The skin under the anode (+) will be dryer and tougher and the burn appears as a hardened lump or scab. It should be treated with care in the same way as above. There are many causes of chemical burns; they are all the result of undue care and lack of attention to detail. Therapists must develop a good technique to avoid these complications.

Accurate technique and careful application will prevent galvanic thermal and chemical burns.

Causes of chemical burns

Chemical burns may occur for the following reasons:

1 If the intensity of the current is too high and if the treatment time is too long – these will cause greater concentrations of both sodium hydroxide at the cathode $(-)$ and hydrochloric acid at the anode $(+)$.

2 If the current concentrates on one area. This may be due to:
   (a) A break in the skin.
   (b) The pads being unevenly folded and of uneven thickness.
   (c) The pads being unevenly moistened or containing undissolved salt.
   (d) The electrode or its connections coming into direct contact with the skin.

3 If the current is applied with metal touching the tissues, either in the form of jewellery, or metal plates and pins in tissues, or IUD coils. Always remove jewellery and avoid giving treatment to areas around metal plates and IUD coils.

4 If the pads are too close so that current concentrates between them.

5 If the pads are too thin, the acid and alkali will not be absorbed and dissipated.

6 If the chemicals have not been washed out of the pads after a previous treatment.

7 If the client has defective skin sensation and is unable to feel that the intensity is too high or that the current is concentrating in one spot.

8 If the treatment has not been explained carefully to the client. (The importance of reporting discomfort and hot spots and the consequences of not doing so must be explained clearly to the client.)

Shock

There is a danger of shock to the client:

1 If the apparatus is faulty and monitoring controls are not functioning and operating correctly.

2 If the current intensity is increased too quickly or reduced suddenly.

3 If skin resistance drops suddenly. As the skin becomes moist, the resistance to the current is lowered. Modern equipment will adjust automatically to a fall in skin resistance and the current intensity will reduce accordingly. However, when using the older constant voltage machines, the current intensity must be reduced manually as the skin resistance falls. Therefore, the apparatus must be checked before treatment.

Precautions

1 Check for contraindications.

2 Test for skin sensitivity.

3 Check that all jewellery has been removed.

4 Wash the area thoroughly.

5 Check the machine and test it on yourself; ensure the intensity controls are at zero.

6 If using a saline solution, mix 2 teaspoonfuls of salt per litre of

warm water; make sure that all the crystals have dissolved.

7 Prepare the pads. They must be of even thickness and not worn or cracked.

(a) Measure the pads to calculate the current intensity, which should be 0.05 mA per square cm.

(b) If using pre-made pads or sponge envelopes, ensure that they are of high density foam at least 1 cm or ½ inch thick.

(c) If using lint pads, carefully fold the sides to middle. Ensure that there are 16 layers and of even thickness, that they are smooth and contain no wrinkles or frayed edges.

(d) Ensure that the pads are 1 cm or ½ inch larger than the electrode all around.

(e) Wash the pads in warm water to make absolutely sure that no chemicals remain in the pads from previous use.

8 Saturate the pads well and evenly. Wet and squeeze out any excess solution.

9 Mould the pad and electrode to the part, cover with insulating fabric and strap evenly and securely; ensure that there are no gaps between the skin and pad.

10 Turn the current up slowly; adjust if necessary.

11 At the end of the treatment, turn the current down slowly.

12 Speak to the client throughout the treatment.

13 Wash the area thoroughly with warm soapy water after treatment to remove chemical build up on the skin.

14 Wash the pads in warm soapy water, rinse and hang to dry.

Figure 8.11   Method of applying lint pad

Figure 8.12   Method of applying sponge envelopes

18 cm × 9 cm = 162 square centimetres
162 × 0.05 = 8.10 milliamps

Figure 8.13 To calculate the intensity of the current required for body treatment measure two sides of the pad (one long and one short) multiply these, to obtain the number of square centimetres. Each square centimetre of pad should receive 0.05 milliamps of current, therefore multiply the number of square centimetres by 0.05 milliamps. Therefore for this size of pad the maximum amperage would be eight milliamps. Manufacturer's usually recommend intensity parameters.

Treatment technique

Preparation of the client

1 Consider the areas to be treated and position the client accordingly. If the thighs and hips are to be treated, place the client in the supine position (face up). If the buttocks or back are to be treated, place the client in the prone position (face down).

2 Check that all jewellery has been removed.

3 Check for contraindications.

4 Check particularly for broken skin (e.g. cuts and abrasions) as it offers low resistance to current, therefore the current would concentrate here and cause a burn. Small cuts can be insulated with petroleum jelly and covered with waterproof plasters.

5 Test skin sensitivity with hot and cold test tubes and a blunt needle and cotton wool (see page 154).

6 Wash the area thoroughly to remove sweat, moisturisers, lotions, perfumes, etc.

7 Explain the treatment to the client.

Procedure

1 Place the machine on a stable base and check that the plugs, electrodes, leads and terminals are sound and secure.

2 Check that the intensity controls are at zero, and if there is a shunt (which multiplies the intensity by ten) move this to the low point.

3 Test the machine.

4 Collect all the prepared items mentioned previously and have them to hand.

5 Wash the pads in warm water and then either wet them in saline solution and squeeze out the excess or, if using gels, etc., soak them with water and squeeze out the excess.

6 If a gel or ampule is used, either apply this directly to the area ensuring an even application, or soak into a piece of gauze and apply this to the skin ensuring a smooth, even contact.

7 Place the electrode over the pad (or in a pouch) making sure than the pad is 1 cm or ½ inch bigger all around, and is 1 cm or ½ inch deep. (The pad must lie between the skin and the electrode.)

8 Place the active electrode over the treatment area and the inactive electrode opposite or parallel to it. Mould them to the body. If using a

saline solution the cathode (−) will be the active electrode. If using products, follow the manufacturer's instructions. If the product contains negative anions, the cathode (−) will be the active electrode, but if the product contains positive cations, the anode (+) will be the active electrode.

9 Cover both electrodes with insulating fabric (rubber, plastic or polythene). There must be no holes in this. This is so that the connective straps do not become conductive.

10 Secure the pad and insulating fabric evenly in position with straps (make sure the electrodes mould to the body and contain no air spaces and that strapping applies even pressure all over).

11 Explain the sensation to the client and stress the importance of reporting any discomfort, any concentration

(a) Full body padding – anterior

(b) Full body padding – posterior

(c) Leg padding – parallel padding

(d) Leg padding – opposite padding

Figure 8.14   a) full body padding – anterior, b) full body padding – posterior, c) leg padding – parallel padding, d) leg padding – opposite padding.

of current in one area or any hot spots. The client should feel a slight tingling sensation which will give way to *mild* warmth.

12 Check that the electrodes have not moved.

13 Turn up the intensity control very slowly until a sensation of warmth is felt. The desired intensity will depend on the client's tolerance, product usage and size of the pad. Most products and client comfort indicate 0.05 mA per sq cm.

14 Stay with the client; as the treatment progresses, the skin resistance will fall. Some machines that are designed as constant voltage will register an increase in intensity as the skin resistance falls. With this type of machine, the intensity will need to be turned down accordingly. Most modern systems are designed as constant current, and will automatically adjust to changes in body resistance.

15 The treatment should last for 20 minutes; at the end of treatment, turn the intensity control down very slowly. (A sudden increase or decrease in current intensity gives the client a shock, as the muscles may contract.)

16 The skin should be evenly pink under each pad, and there should be a more marked reaction under the cathode (−).

17 If using saline, wash the skin thoroughly with warm, soapy water and dry gently. This will remove any acid or alkali. Apply a soothing lotion or talc.

18 Wash the pads thoroughly in soapy water, rinse and leave them to dry.

Do not carry out any other treatment over the area of the skin under the pads, as it is very sensitive.

REMEMBER! Feedback and after care.

Combined systems

Body wraps, clays, combined EMS and galvanic treatments

These treatments require specialized tuition from the manufacturers as each system differs in terms of application. Therapists must ensure that they attend courses and read the manufacturer's instructions carefully before embarking on these treatments.

Figure 8.15   Client receiving body wrap treatment

SUMMARY

- Galvanic treatments use a low voltage direct (or constant) current, sometimes called a galvanic current. This current flows in one direction only and has polarity.
- One electrode is negatively charged, called the cathode; the other electrode is positively charged, called the anode.
- Treatments which use the direct current are:
  (a) **Disincrustation** – facial treatment – cleansing.
  (b) **Iontophoresis** – facial treatment – beneficial ions for various skin types.
  (c) **Body galvanism** – body cellulite using sodium chloride solution.
  (d) **Body iontophoresis** – body cellulite using products.
- There is a variety of other body systems utilizing clays, wraps, etc. (epilation is not covered in this book.)
- The effects produced depend on two scientific principles: the chemistry of electrolysis, and the law of physics which states that like charges repel (i.e. positive repels positive and negative repels negative) and opposite charges attract (i.e. positive attracts negative).
- An electrolyte is a chemical compound which transmits a current. It may be a solution or paste. The compounds making up the solution dissociate (split) into cations (+) and anions (−). These move towards opposite poles because of the attraction of opposite charges. Therefore: *cations* (+) move towards the *cathode* (−), and *anions* (−) move towards the *anode* (+). Certain chemical reactions take place at the electrodes.
- When using sodium chloride solution (salt and water), the reactions at the electrodes will produce: sodium hydroxide (alkali) and hydrogen gas at the cathode and hydrochloric acid and oxygen gas at the anode.

Disincrustation treatment to the face

- This uses lint soaked in sodium chloride or other products over the active electrode. When the current is flowing, the alkali, sodium hydroxide, is produced at the cathode. This alkali will saponify sebum, break down keratin and relax pores, releasing blockages and sebum which will soften and cleanse the skin.
- Its disadvantages are that it has a very drying effect and that it destroys the acid mantle. If the polarity is reversed at the end of the treatment, the hydrochloric acid produced restores the acid mantle.

Iontophoresis

- This is the repulsion of ions of beneficial substances into the skin. These substances must be placed under the correct electrode for repulsion to take place.

summary continues overleaf

summary continued from previous page

If the product contains negative anions, the negative cathode must be used for repulsion (anion active). If the product contains positive cations, the positive anode must be used for repulsion (cation active). Remember, like charges repel.

■ This is a very effective and useful treatment as a wide variety of products are available to treat most skin types.

■ There is very little danger with facial work, as the current intensities are low and the electrodes are moving. However, the client will receive a shock if the intensity is turned up or down too quickly, or if the electrode is lifted off the skin with the intensity turned up. This is because the sudden surge of current will stimulate the muscles to contract.

■ The intensity of the current used for facial work will depend on the tolerance of the client and the erythema reaction produced. From 0.05–2 mA maximum is recommended by most manufacturers.

■ It is essential to establish that the client is able to feel heat or sharp touch so that she can report any feeling of discomfort (for both facial and body work). Failure to report these sensations may result in burns. Test over the area receiving treatment with a hot and a cold test tube and with sharp and blunt instruments (an orange stick and some cotton wool are suitable). The client must close her eyes and identify which item is in contact with her skin.

Body galvanism

■ This uses pads soaked in saline solution. The active electrode is the cathode (−). The inactive electrode is placed opposite it or parallel with it.

■ The effects are produced by the formation of irritating sodium hydroxide and hydrogen at the cathode and by changes in circulation, metabolic rate and water content of the tissue through which the current passes. It is used to reduce and soften areas of cellulite.

Body iontophoresis

■ This uses a gel or liquid anti-cellulite preparation placed under the appropriate electrode: negative under the cathode and positive under the anode. This substance will be repelled into the skin to produce the desired effect. There will also be changes in the circulation and metabolic rate of the tissue through which the current passes.

Body systems which apply specially manufactured serums, etc., via wraps and clays to the whole or large parts of the body

■ These use very low intensity current to stimulate the circulation.

Dangers

■ Chemical burns, thermal burns and electric shock.

summary continues overleaf

summary continued from previous page

Check list

All students should ensure that they have checked and carried out all the following points of technique.

1   Make the client comfortable in a suitable position.
2   Remove all jewellery, any metal or water from the area.
3   Test for skin sensitivity – hot/cold; blunt/sharp.
4   Check for contraindications.
5   Wash the area thoroughly.
6   Check that the machine and all plugs, leads, electrodes and terminals are sound and secure.
7   Ensure that the intensity controls are at zero.
8   Prepare the pads, ensuring that they are:
    (a) Of even texture and density.
    (b) Folded evenly – no wrinkles or frayed edges.
    (c) 1 cm or ½ inch thick, 1 cm or ½ inch larger than the electrode all around.
9   Mix a saline solution: 2 teaspoons of salt to 1 litre of warm water. Make sure all the salt has dissolved.
10 Wet pads and squeeze out the excess. If using a gel or lotion, soak a piece of gauze or apply thinly and evenly over the skin under active electrode.
11 Select the cathode (−) as the active electrode and the anode (+) as the inactive electrode (unless the product carries a positive charge).
12 Position the pad, electrode and waterproof insulating fabric.
13 Secure evenly and firmly with strapping; mould to the part leaving no air gaps.
14 Explain the sensation and impress upon the client the importance of reporting any discomfort.
15 Turn the current intensity up *slowly*; watch the milliammeter and the client. (The intensity must be within the tolerance of the client – around 0.05 mA per sq cm of pad).
16 Stay with the client and turn down the intensity as the skin resistance falls if the machine does not automatically adjust.
17 At the end of the treatment time, approximately 20 minutes, turn the intensity down *slowly*.
18 Remove the pads.
19 Examine and wash the area thoroughly – apply talc or lotion.
20 Do not carry out further treatments over the area of skin under electrodes as it is very sensitive.
21 Wash the pads thoroughly, rinse and dry them.

summary continues overleaf

summary continued from previous page

Feedback

Examine the area and ask appropriate questions to obtain feedback; this will indicate if the treatment is effective and suitable and the client is happy.

After care

Give advice on immediate feedback and any routine to follow before the next treatment.

QUESTIONS

1   Galvanic treatments use a direct current; explain briefly what is meant by direct current.

2   List the four treatments that use the direct current.

3   A direct current has polarity; give the name and charge of each pole.

4   When the compound sodium chloride dissolves in water it ionizes into two ions; name the two ions and give their charge.

5   When a direct current is passed through saline (salt) solution, name:

   (a) The alkali formed under the cathode.

   (b) The acid formed under the anode.

6   Explain the terms 'active electrode' and 'inactive electrode'.

7   Which electrode would be selected as the active electrode for disincrustation treatments using a salt solution?

8   Give the skin type suitable for disincrustation treatments.

9   Explain briefly why the polarity of the electrodes may be changed for 2–5 minutes at the end of disincrustation treatment.

10   Give the physical theories on which the treatment of iontophoresis depends.

11   Explain why the choice of products is very important when using iontophoresis treatments.

12   Give four contraindications to facial galvanic treatments.

13   Give the function of the milliammeter.

14   How is the milliammeter calibrated?

15   On what factor does the selection of current intensity depend? Indicate the maximum current for facial work.

16   Body galvanism is given to improve areas of hard fat or cellulite. Give two reasons why it is effective.

questions continues overleaf

questions continued from previous page

17   Why do thin or uneven pads constitute a danger to the client?

18   Explain the importance of dissolving all the crystals of salt.

19   Why should one carry out a skin sensitivity test?

20   Explain the procedure for testing skin sensitivity.

21   Explain why the skin and the pads should be thoroughly washed after each treatment.

22   Why might the current intensity increase slightly at the beginning of treatment although the control is not moved?

23   Explain the action to be taken if the current intensity increases (on older machines).

24   How would you instruct the client at commencement of treatment?

25   Briefly explain why the skin will be red at the end of a treatment.

Oral questions

Facial galvanic treatment: disincrustation

1   What type of current is used in disincrustation treatment?

2   Give two very important procedures which must be carried out prior to treatment.

3   Why is careful skin analysis important prior to disincrustation treatment?

4   Why is the skin sensitivity test so important?

5   Why might the client have difficulty in detecting heat and sharp objects?

6   If the client was unable to tell which was hot or cold, sharp or blunt, what procedure should you follow?

7   Why would you select disincrustation treatment for use on a client?

8   What products would you use for disincrustation?

9   How is the current applied to the client?

10   Why did you place lint/sponge covers on the electrodes?

11   How does the treatment cleanse the skin?

12   (a) Are there any undesirable effects to the treatment?

     (b) Can this be rectified?

13   What is the timing of this treatment?

14   What procedure do you follow before turning the current on?

15   Why is it important to place the active electrode on a sensitive area when turning up the intensity?

16   Why is it important to turn the current intensity up slowly?

17   What intensity of current would you select?

18   Why is it necessary to place petroleum jelly under the eye area?

questions continues overleaf

questions continued from previous page

Facial galvanic treatment: iontophoresis

1   What current is used for iontophoresis?
2   How is the current applied to the client?
3   Which electrode would be the active electrode?
4   Why is the selection of the correct electrode important?
5   What type of client would benefit from iontophoresis?
6   How does this treatment improve the skin?
7   How did you select current intensity?
8   How long would you give the treatment?

Body galvanic treatments

1   What type of current is used in body galvanic treatment?
2   What type of client would benefit from galvanic treatment?
3   How is the client prepared for treatment?
4   How is the current delivered to the client.
5   Why is it important to evenly cover the electrodes?
6   (a) Explain what happens under the cathode (polar effect at cathode).
     (b) Explain what happens under the anode.
7   Does anything happen in the tissues between the electrodes/poles (interpolar effects)?
8   What are the reasons for taking great care when giving galvanic treatments?
9   Is there a danger of shock? How would you avoid this?
10   How would you deal with any burn?
11   What intensity of current would you use?
12   How long a treatment would you give?
13   Why is it necessary to place the client in a prone lying position when treating the posterior aspect of the body?
14   What is body iontophoresis?

9 Muscle Stimulation and Microcurrent Treatment

OBJECTIVES

After you have studied this chapter you will be able to:

1 Describe the structure of skeletal muscle tissue.

2 List the parts of the nervous system.

3 Differentiate between sensory, motor and connector neurones.

4 Explain the nature and transmission of a nerve impulse.

5 Describe the 'motor unit'.

6 Draw a diagram to illustrate the pathway of an impulse from the brain to a muscle fibre.

7 Differentiate between muscle fibre types and their stimulation by specific frequencies.

8 Describe the type of current and wave forms used for muscle stimulation.

9 List the factors that influence the response of the muscle.

10 Identify the position of the motor points of the superficial muscles of the body.

11 Explain the three different methods of padding.

12 Select suitable patterns of padding to suit the needs of the client.

13 Identify the controls on the machine and explain their effects.

14 Identify the contraindications to treatment.

15 Apply pads accurately and securely to the body.

16 Select the appropriate parameters to suit the needs of the client.

17 Treat the client, paying due consideration to maximum efficiency, comfort, safety and hygiene.

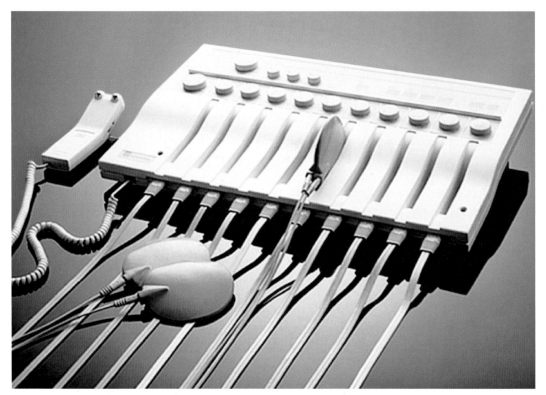

Figure 9.1   Electronic unit for muscle stimulation

Electrical Stimulation of Muscles

Figure 9.1 is a photograph of a modern, sophisticated electronic machine used for muscle stimulation. A variety of muscle stimulators are to be found on the market, and they range from simple single outlet machines with pre-set controls to the very complex machines with multi-outlets and a range of variable controls. However, they all produce electrical pulses which are applied to the body by means of electrodes. When the pulses are applied, they stimulate the motor nerves and result in the contraction of muscles. The muscles are made to contract and relax, simulating active exercise. The treatment is used to improve muscle tone and condition and to maintain muscle strength.

The impulses are produced by modifying direct or alternating currents. The current amplitude must be variable and must be of sufficient intensity and duration to produce a contraction.

Normal muscle contraction is brought about when impulses from the brain are transmitted via motor nerves to the muscles. The impulses produced by machines have the same effect as those from the brain. They stimulate the motor nerve directly and this will initiate a contraction in the muscles supplied by that nerve (see page 181).

To produce a contraction, the current must be variable; it must be of high enough intensity; it must be of sufficient duration.

The original current used for muscle stimulation was produced by the Smart-Bristow coil and was known as the **faradic current**. This term is sometimes used today to describe muscle-stimulating treatments (e.g. faradism or faradic treatment). Manufacturers' names are also used to describe the treatments, for example, Ultratone, Slendertone, Slim-line and others. The terms TENS, EMS and NMES (NMS) are also used.

- TENS stands for transcutaneous electrical nerve stimulation. This type of stimulation is used for pain control and is not generally used in beauty therapy. Modern equipment may include TENS to reduce pain and therefore improve client comfort.

- EMS stands for electrical muscle stimulation. This term covers stimulation of both innervated muscle and denervated muscle – innervated muscle refers to muscle with an intact nerve supply whilst denervated muscle means one lacking in nerve supply due to injury or disease. Different types of pulses are used for these two types of muscle.

- NMES or NMS stands for neuromuscular (electrical) stimulation. This term covers the stimulation of innervated muscle. The pulse is used to stimulate a nerve and the impulse is transmitted via the nerve to the muscle, initiating a contraction. When using nerve stimulation to produce muscle contraction, it is more accurate to use the terms NMES or NMS when referring to these treatments. However, EMS is commonly used.

- MES stands for microcurrent electrical stimulation. The muscle fibres are stimulated directly by very low amperage current.

Underpinning Knowledge

Nerve–muscle physiology

This section explains the relationship between nerve impulses and muscle contraction. The voluntary contraction of skeletal muscle is controlled by the brain. Impulses initiated in the brain are transmitted via the spinal cord and peripheral motor nerve to the muscle fibres, causing them to contract. Electrical pulses imitate these impulses.

Skeletal muscle

Skeletal muscle is composed of long, thin, multinucleated cells called muscle fibres. These muscle fibres are composed of myofibrils separated by sarcoplasm, and they have an outer membrane called the sarcolemma. Muscle fibres are grouped together to form muscle bundles, and many bundles make up the complete muscle. Under an electron microscope, light and dark bands can be seen along the length of the fibre; these are known as A and I bands and are composed of two types of protein: actin and myosin. The movement of these bands into each other constitutes muscle contraction.

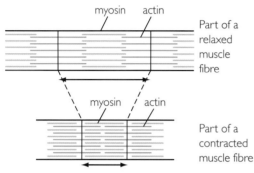

Figure 9.2   Relaxed and contracted muscle fibres

> The best contraction is obtained when the pad is placed on the motor point. This is where the nerve enters the belly of the muscle.

Muscles will contract in response to stimuli. Normally, these stimuli originate in the brain and are transmitted to muscle fibres via nerves. Because the stimuli are electrical in nature, a suitable electrical pulse from a machine can be used to initiate a contraction. The electrical pulse can be applied anywhere along the course of a motor nerve, but the best response is obtained if it is applied at the point where the nerve enters the belly of the muscle, known as the motor point. Each muscle fibre is sensitive to impulses reaching it from the central nervous system.

The nervous system

The system is made up of:

1   The central nervous system comprising the brain and the spinal cord.

2   The peripheral nervous system comprising:
    (a) Twelve pairs of cranial nerves arising from the brain.
    (b) Thirty-one pairs of spinal nerves arising from the spinal cord.

3   The autonomic system.

Nervous tissue is composed of the functional units which conduct impulses, called **neurones,** and the supporting tissue, called **neuroglia**. There are three types of neurones:

1   Sensory neurones (or nerves): these carry impulses from the sensory organs to the spinal cord and brain.

2   Motor neurones: these carry impulses away from the brain and spinal cord to muscles and glands.

3   Connector neurones or interneurones: these are found in the brain and spinal cord and form connections between neurones.

Neurones are similar in structure having a cell body and two types of processes called axons and dendrons.

- Axons carry impulses *away* from the cell body.

- Dendrons carry impulses *towards* the cell body.

- Dendrons have small terminal branches called *dendrites*.

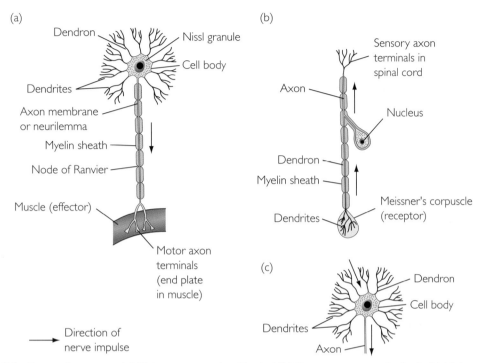

Figure 9.3   Types of neurones (a) Motor neurones (multipolar) (b) Sensory neurones (unipolar) (c) Interneurone (stellate)

The transmission of nerve impulses

Impulses are transmitted in axons and dendrons in one direction only. Impulses move along a nerve because of a change in its electrically charged state. This is brought about by the movement of positive and negative ions across the nerve membrane.

When the nerve membrane is at rest, solutions of sodium chloride, potassium chloride and various proteins are found inside and outside the membrane. The salts ionize in solution giving sodium (+) ions and chloride (−) ions outside, with potassium (+) ions and chloride (−) ions inside, together with non-diffusable anions and negative proteins, inside the membrane which maintain the negative potential across the membrane.

When the nerve membrane is non-conductive, there are more positive ions outside and more negative ions inside. Therefore a potential difference exists across the membrane. In this state of rest, the nerve is said to be **polarized.**

When a stimulus is applied to the nerve, the following reactions will occur: there will be a fall of potential difference across the membrane; the permeability of the membrane changes; the diffusable ions move across the membrane until the polarity is reversed, that is there will be more negative ions outside and more positive ions inside. The nerve is now said to be **depolarized.**

When the concentration of ions reaches a certain level, the positive sodium ions are 'pumped out' and the nerve returns to its resting state, that is it is repolarized. This change of state occurs along the nerve and constitutes the passage of the impulse.

■ The impulse leaves A and is transmitted to B when the polarity is reversed. The impulse will move along when the polarity returns to normal at B but is reversed at C. The impulse is thus transmitted along the nerve fibre.

■ More than one neurone will be involved in the transmission of a nerve impulse.

■ Neurones do not connect directly with each other – there is always a gap between the end of one neurone and the beginning of another. This is known as a synapse.

■ There are similar specialized synapses between motor neurones and muscle fibres known as the neuro-muscular junction. The impulse is transmitted across the gap by the chemical transmitter acetylcholine.

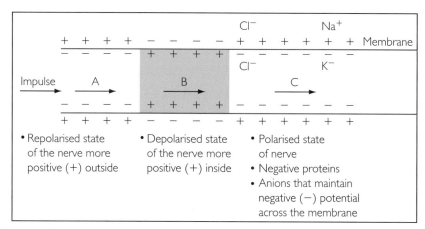

Figure 9.4   Passage of a nerve impulse along an axon

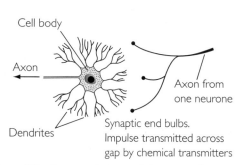

Figure 9.5   Synapse between interconnecting neurones

Figure 9.6   Synapse between nerve terminal and muscle fibre

Pathway of an impulse

An impulse initiated in the cells of the motor cortex of the brain will be transmitted via the axon (of the upper motor neurone) to the anterior/ventral horn of the spinal cord. Here the impulse will cross a synapse to stimulate the cell of another neurone (the lower motor neurone) to be transmitted via its axon to the muscle fibre.

Each anterior/ventral horn cell has one axon which leaves the spinal cord by the anterior/ventral root. The axons of many cells will emerge together as a motor nerve and pass to a muscle where they will enter at the **motor point.**

Each axon will then divide into many branches or terminals (from 5–150) depending on the function of the muscle. Muscles requiring fine control have smaller motor units with fewer branches and can, therefore, produce more finely graded movements.

Each axon branch will supply one muscle fibre. The junction between the axon branch and the muscle fibre is known as the neuro-muscular junction. Here the ends of the axons expand a little into bulbs; they approach but do not contact the muscle fibre. There is always a gap in between called a synapse. The sarcolemma covering the muscle fibre is modified at this point and is known as the **motor end plate.**

The anterior horn cell, the axon, axon branches and the muscle fibres they supply make up the **motor unit.**

> **Motor point** – where the nerve enters the belly of the muscle.

This is not only an anatomical unit but also a functional unit. Impulses generated at the anterior horn cell will pass via the axon to all the fibres supplied by the axon branches and all those fibres will contract simultaneously. The frequency of the impulses passing along the nerve will determine the strength of contraction in each motor unit.

During voluntary movement, motor units work an on/off 'shift' system. Some will contract while others will be at rest. When a stronger contraction is required, more motor units are activated. The frequency and number of motor units activated will determine the strength of contraction of the whole muscle.

> **Motor unit** – this includes the anterior horn cell, the axon, the axon branches and the muscle fibres supplied by each branch.

Muscle fibre types

A muscle is composed of different types of muscle fibres. This enables individual muscles to perform various functions. Research has shown that these differences are imposed upon the fibres by their motor neurones. By imposing a certain pattern of activity on to the fibre, different physiological and biochemical properties develop. All the muscle fibres supplied by one motor neurone have similar properties.

Impulses from the central nervous system (CNS), which stimulate the different muscle fibres, are discharged at different frequencies.

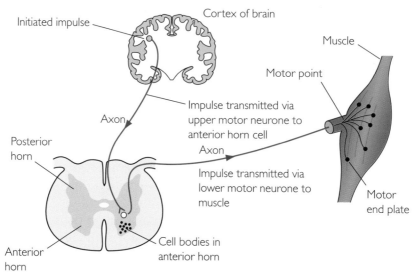

Initiated impulse

Cortex of brain

Muscle

Motor point

Axon

Impulse transmitted via upper motor neurone to anterior horn cell

Posterior horn

Axon

Impulse transmitted via lower motor neurone to muscle

Motor end plate

Anterior horn

Cell bodies in anterior horn

Figure 9.7   Pathway of an impulse from brain to muscle fibre

Frequency means the number of pulses per second.

This becomes an important consideration when using electrical stimulation. Selection of the appropriate frequencies must be made for effective stimulation of the whole muscle. Specific frequencies can be used to produce certain characteristics in fibres when training athletes for particular events.

Properties of muscle fibres

- **Slow oxidative fibres (SO)**, red fibres or slow twitch fibres: These fibres are capable of sustaining tension for long periods, and are active for nearly 24 hours per day. They have a high level of endurance without fatigue. Containing high levels of oxidative enzymes, they depend mainly on aerobic metabolism. They are well supplied with blood having a high-density capillary network. They are recruited for endurance activities, such as maintenance of posture, swimming and marathon running. Certain muscles will have a much higher proportion of these fibres (e.g. the soleus muscle). Impulses are transmitted to these fibres at frequencies of between 6 and 15 Hz.

- **Fast glycolytic fibres (FG)**, white fibres or fast twitch fibres: These fibres are used intermittently for short periods only. They are recruited when speed, e.g. reflex activity and burst of power are required. They have low levels of endurance and fatigue easily. They have high levels of glycolytic enzymes and depend on anaerobic metabolism; they have a low-density capillary network. Certain muscles will have high proportions of these fibres, e.g. the orbital muscles of the eye, *orbicularis oculi*. Impulses are transmitted to these fibres at frequencies of between 30 and 80 Hz.

- **Fast oxidative glycolytic (FOG)** fibres: These are used for around 60 per cent of the day. They contain both oxidative and glycolytic enzymes and are recruited for general activities that require neither speed nor endurance. Impulses are transmitted to these fibres at frequencies of between 20 and 40 Hz.

A muscle will be composed of a mixture of fibres – the percentage of each fibre type will differ for each muscle and will depend on the function of the muscle. Research has shown that electrical stimulation can be used to change muscle properties.

If fast glycolytic muscle fibres are stimulated at frequencies between 6 and 15 Hz on a daily basis for a considerable length of time, they contract more slowly and do not fatigue easily. The biochemical characteristics are also changed; there is a decrease in glycolytic enzymes and an increase in oxidative enzymes; capillary density also increases. Thus fast glycolytic fibres can be changed to slow oxidative fibres (SO fibres do not respond in the same way).

This ability to change muscle fibre type is used medically (when a muscle has been transplanted and is required to change its function (e.g. replacing sphincters and cardiac assistance in heart disease).

Electrical stimulation

As explained above, a muscle will contract in response to an impulse from the brain, reaching it via its motor nerve. Stimuli or pulses of current produced by machines and applied to the motor nerve by electrodes will produce the same result, that is contraction of muscles supplied by that nerve.

Modern units which produce these pulses are very sophisticated electronic units. (The older faradic current has now largely been replaced by interrupted direct current.)

> EMS units produce interrupted direct current of low frequency around 10–120 Hz.

Some foreign units use modified AC, but British units in the main use modified DC. These units produce low frequency, interrupted direct current of between 10 and 120 Hz. There are units on the market which offer upper range low frequency current of between 200 and 800 Hz. Research has shown, however, that maximal force is developed in human muscle at between 40 and 80 Hz. There is, therefore, little purpose in using higher frequencies, and careful consideration should be given to the effects of using these frequencies. Although sensory stimulation is reduced by higher frequencies, and they 'feel more comfortable', their safety and some of the claims made should be questioned as the mode in which they work is unclear.

Although there are a large number of different units available, one basic concept remains common to all – impulses are produced which stimulate the motor nerves resulting in the contraction of muscles supplied by those nerves. The muscles are made to actively contract and then relax, improving their tone and condition and maintaining strength, providing that the treatment is carried out on a regular basis.

Pulses, impulses and stimuli

- A constant flow of current or a slow, rising electrical pulse will not produce a contraction as the muscle adapts to the current. This is known as accommodation.

- The direct current must be modified to produce pulses which rise steeply and fall at regular intervals.

- The intensity must be high enough and the duration of the pulse long enough to produce a contraction.

- I is the intensity of the current; on the machine this is controlled by the intensity control to each pair of electrodes.

- D is the duration of the pulse or pulse width; this is pre-set on some machines but others have a pulse width control. A pulse width of under 100 microamps (μs) is not effective

and the best results are obtained with pulse widths of between 200 and 300 μs.

- Some units produce pulses of different shapes.

- The shape of the pulse is known as the wave form (see Figure 9.9).

- It is the rate of rise of each pulse that determines the response in the muscle. A pulse which rises sharply produces the best response in innervated muscle and the rectangular pulse is generally used in beauty therapy units.

- A single, adequate pulse will produce a twitch in the muscle. The muscle contracts as the current rises and the contraction diminishes as the current falls; the muscle relaxes completely when the current stops.

- If a number of pulses are applied to the muscle, the type of contraction produced will depend on the interval between the pulses.

- If the interval between pulses is long enough for the muscle to relax, then a series of twitches will be produced in the muscle, giving a tremulous contraction.

Sharply rising pulse

Slow rising pulse

Figure 9.8   Sharp and slow rising pulses

- If the pulses follow each other in rapid succession, the muscle has no time to relax and a smooth contraction is produced. A smooth contraction of a muscle is known as a **tetanic** contraction.

- The number of pulses produced every second is known as the frequency and is measured in Hz.

> **Wave form** means the shape of the pulse. A rectangular pulse which rises sharply produces the best response in normal muscle.

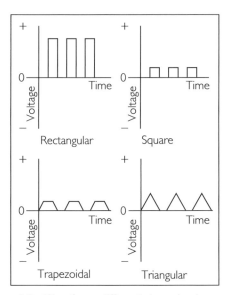

Figure 9.9 Waveform: different shaped pulses

Frequency

- The frequency of the pulses is an important consideration because the different fibres within a muscle will respond in a different way to various frequencies.

- Below 20 Hz (i.e. pulses per second) only the slow fibres will be showing smooth, fused tetanic contractions; the faster fibres will be showing unfused contractions.

- As the frequency is increased to 40 Hz, the majority of fibres will be showing fused tetanic contractions, although some fast fibres may require higher frequencies to produce maximum force.

- At 60 Hz, the majority of fast fibres will be showing smooth, fused tetanic contractions and the whole muscle will contract smoothly. This can be represented diagramatically (Figure 9.11).

- In most human muscle, maximal force is developed in the frequency range of 40–80 Hz, and there is nothing to be gained by using higher frequencies. The highest frequency recorded during normal transmission is around 100 Hz.

Contraction time

- The pulses are grouped together in 'trains' or 'envelopes', with a rest

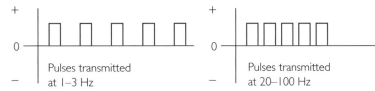

Figure 9.10 Pulses of different frequency

Frequency

20 Hz   Only slow fibres show fused contractions and the muscle contraction is not smooth

40 Hz   The majority of fibres show fused contractions and the muscle contraction becomes smoother

60 Hz   All fibres showing smooth, fused contraction and the muscle contraction is very smooth

Figure 9.11   Muscle contraction at different frequency

period in between. When the current flows, the muscle contracts; when the current stops, the muscle relaxes.

- On most machines, the contraction and relaxation period can be varied.

- In order to improve client comfort, the pulse envelope is surged so that

Pulse envelope or train

C is the contraction time
R is the relaxation time

Figure 9.12   Trains or envelopes of pulses

the strength of the pulses rises gradually to peak intensity.

- The current may then stop suddenly on some units, or decrease gradually on others.

- The rate of rise of the current is known as the ramp time.

Phasic selection

- Many units have a phasic control and offer a choice of monophasic or biphasic current.

- With monophasic current, the current flows mainly in one direction, that is electrons flow from the negative electrode (cathode) to the positive electrode (anode) without variation.

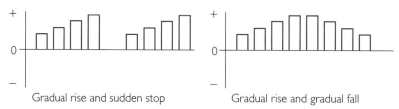

Gradual rise and sudden stop   Gradual rise and gradual fall

Figure 9.13   Surged envelopes

Consequently, the negative electrode will produce the stronger contraction. This is an important consideration when using duplicate or split padding. The negative electrode (cathode) should always be placed on the weaker muscle or weaker side and should also be used as the mushroom electrode for the stimulation of individual muscles, the indifferent anode being placed elsewhere.

■ With biphasic current, each alternate pulse is reversed so that with the first pulse, electron flow is from cathode to anode but the second pulse flow is reversed. In this way polarity is cancelled out and even strength contractions are produced under each pad.

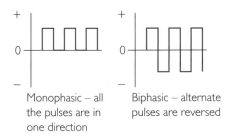

Figure 9.14   Monophasic and biphasic pulses

Types of electrodes

The current is conducted from the machine to the client by means of leads and electrodes. These electrodes come in various forms:

1   **Rubber pads** These are the most common form of electrode. They are made of rubber impregnated with a good conductor, such as graphite. They come in various sizes and may be round or square. Only one side is conductive, the other side is rubber insulated.

2   **Metal plates** These are no longer used with modern equipment. They are made of tin, cut to the required size and attached to the lead with a clip. They were placed on top of 16 layers of lint.

3   **Mushroom or disc electrodes** These are metal discs on the end of wooden handles. The discs are covered with 16 layers of lint. They are useful for individual stimulation of small muscles.

4   **Facial block electrode** This has both electrodes, the anode and cathode, set into an insulating holder. It is used to stimulate facial muscles.

5   **Facial mask electrode** This has many electrodes fitted into the mask. It covers the face and stimulates the muscles simultaneously.

6   **Roller electrodes** These are small metal cylinders covered with lint.

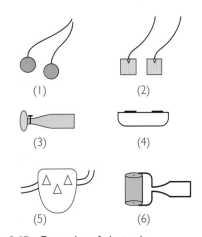

Figure 9.15   Examples of electrodes

They are used for labile treatments on large sheets of muscle, such as the back muscles. The roller is moved slowly over the back stimulating the muscles as it passes over the motor points.

Facial muscles

Muscle	Position	Action
Occipito frontalis	Covers top of skull	Wrinkles the forehead, raises the eyebrows, moves the scalp
Corrugator	Between the eyebrows	Draws eyebrows inwards and down
Nasalis	Side of nose	Compresses the nostrils
Orbicularis oculi	Surrounds the eye	Closes the eye gently or tightly
Levators of the upper lip	Above the upper lip	Raises the upper lip
Zygomaticus	Above the corner of the mouth to zygmatic bone	Raises the corner of the mouth
Buccinator	Deep, horizontal in the cheek	Draws the cheek towards the teeth when chewing
Masseter	Between mandible and zygomatic arch	Raises the mandible to close the mouth
Depressor anguli oris	Below corner of the mouth	Draws corner of the mouth downwards
Orbicularis oris	Around the mouth	Closes and protrudes the lips
Digastric	Beneath the chin	Protrudes the jaw, depresses the mandible
Platysma	Covers the side and the front of neck	Depresses the angle of mouth, wrinkles the skin of the neck

Stimulation of the Facial Muscles

This treatment is used to improve facial contours and delay the appearance of ageing. The units for facial stimulation are very simple units with an on/off switch and an intensity control to one pair of electrodes; some have a surge control. Some of the large body units include a special terminal for facial stimulation.

Methods of application

1 **Disc electrode** This is a metal disc covered with 16 layers of lint; it has a wooden handle. This electrode is placed on the motor point of the muscle and is known as the active electrode; a plate electrode, which is placed behind the shoulder or strapped to the arms, is known as the inactive electrode. Specific muscles are stimulated in turn, six to eight contractions per muscle. The procedure is repeated three times.

2 **Facial electrode** Here a plastic or rubber holder contains both the active and the inactive electrode. It is placed over a group of muscles or a branch of the facial nerve, and these are stimulated six to eight times and repeated three times. This method does not produce specific movement of individual muscles, but the simultaneous contractions of many muscles.

3 **Facial mask** Here there are electrodes within a mask which is placed over the face. The muscles are stimulated simultaneously. Modern units have small adhesive electrodes placed on motor points. These are less claustrophobic.

Uses

1 Ageing skin – wrinkled with poor elasticity.

2 Loss of firm contours due to muscle weakness.

3 As a preventative measure to delay the effects of ageing and promote cellular function.

4 Slight puffiness around the eyes.

Effects

1 It improves muscle tone and the general condition of the muscle. This results in improvement of the contours of the face.

2 The pumping action increases the supply of blood to the skin and muscle, thus bringing nutrients and oxygen to the body part and removing waste products. This results in improved condition of skin and muscle.

3 Vasodilation giving erythema.

4 The contraction and relaxation of muscles aids the removal of fluid from the area; it relieves swelling, but this will be temporary.

5 It irritates sensory nerve endings.

Contraindications

1 Highly strung or nervous client.

2 Hypersensitive skins (the current will irritate the skin further).

3 Highly vascular complexions (e.g. rosacea).

4 High blood pressure.

5 Sinus congestion.

6 Headaches or migraine.

7 Many skin abrasions.

8 Over superficial bony areas.

9 Large number of fillings or bridgework.

10 Epileptic or diabetic client.

Precautions

1 Check that all jewellery has been removed.

2 Check for contraindications.

3 Cleanse the skin.

4 Test the current on yourself. Ensure that the machine is stable and safe.

5 If there is a surge control, select the correct length of surge to suit the client (longer surge for poor muscle tone).

6 Ensure that the intensity controls are at zero.

7 Dampen pads with saline and ensure that they remain moist throughout the treatment.

8 Turn up during surge only when the light is on; the client must be able to feel the current increasing and tell you if it becomes uncomfortable.

9 Always turn off before moving the electrode.

10 Do not over treat – six to eight contractions per muscle are required and repeated three times.

11 Treat both sides of the face equally.

> Do not move the electrode with the intensity turned up.

Treatment technique

Preparation of the client

1 Place the client in a well-supported comfortable position.

2 Check that all jewellery has been removed.

3 Cleanse the face thoroughly – tone the skin to remove all grease as this is a barrier to the current.

4 Check for contraindications, particularly for any abrasions, and cover these with petroleum jelly or plaster.

5 Explain the treatment to the client, that is a prickling sensation giving way to contraction. Ask the client to report any discomfort.

Procedure

1 Prepare the machine, place it on a stable base and check that the plugs and leads are secure.

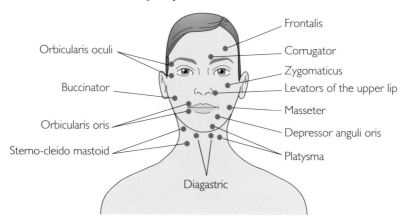

Figure 9.16 Superficial facial muscles

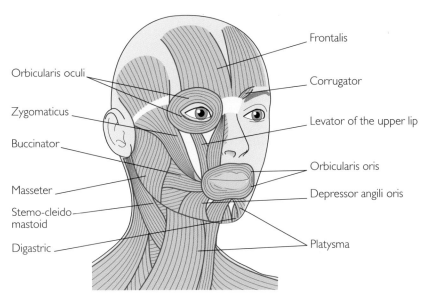

Figure 9.17   Motor points of facial muscles

2 Check that the intensity controls are at zero.

3 Collect commodities: hot water or saline solution and cotton wool.

4 Prepare the electrodes; select the cathode as the active disc electrode (cover them with 16 layers of lint if necessary).

5 Moisten the electrode cover.

6 Check the current on yourself (hold both electrodes in one hand).

7 Turn the dials back to zero.

8 If using a single disc electrode, strap the indifferent electrode behind the shoulder.

9 Place the electrode in position on the face.

10 Tell the client that the machine is being switched on.

11 Turn up the intensity control slowly during the surge until a prickling sensation is felt; continue increasing the intensity until a contraction is obtained.

12 After six to eight contractions, turn the intensity down to zero.

13 Move the electrode to the next muscle and repeat the procedure. Repeat three times.

14 If using a mask or small adhesive electrode, treat the client for 10–15 minutes.

15 When the treatment is complete, turn the intensity to zero, remove the electrode and switch the machine off.

16 Wipe toner over the treated area.

17 Advise on facial exercises for home care.

18 Remove and dispose of lint cover, wipe the electrode with disinfectant wipe.

19 Treatment time 10–15 minutes.

Reasons for poor contractions

1 The intensity is too low (not enough current to initiate a contraction).

2 The pads are too dry or dirty (wet, clean pads are better conductors of current; dirty pads offer resistance).

3 Grease on the skin (grease is a barrier to the current).

4 Incorrect positioning of the pads or mask (padding accurately over the motor point gives the best contraction as this is the point of maximum excitability).

5 Poor contact between the skin and the electrode (gaps offer resistance to current).

6 Poor contact or loose terminals (the current will not flow if the circuit is broken).

NOTE!

1 Talk to the client and reassure her during the treatment.

2 Always turn up the intensity during the surge period.

3 Do not over treat as this will cause muscle fatigue.

4 The therapist should be able to see the machine and the client at all times, and be in easy reach of controls.

5 Check for contra-actions, if there are any stop the treatment.

REMEMBER! Feedback and after care.

Stimulation of Superficial Body Muscles

Figure 9.18   Body electrical treatment

This treatment is used to improve body contours and restore muscle tone. The units for body muscle stimulation are very complex and they have multiple outlets. The controls vary in number and in terminology. The therapist must familiarize herself with the machines she is using in order to select the settings to suit the client.

The rest period must be equal to or longer than the surge period to prevent muscle fatigue.

Machine controls

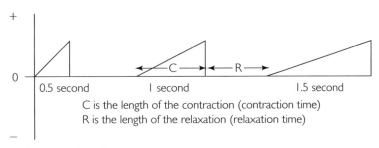

C is the length of the contraction (contraction time)
R is the length of the relaxation (relaxation time)

Figure 9.19   Surges of different length

1 **On/off switch** This switches the current on and off; there is usually a light which comes on to show that the current is flowing.

2 **Surge control/surge envelope/contraction time/stimulation period** This controls the length of time the current is flowing, that is the length of the surge envelope or train; it controls the length of time the muscle contracts. While the current flows, the muscle contracts; when the current stops, the muscle relaxes. The surge length should be long enough to produce a good contraction. Muscles with poor tone or with a thick layer of covering fat require a longer surge. The surge control usually varies from ½ second to 2½ seconds.

3 **Relaxation control/interval or rest period** This controls the length of the rest period between the contractions. The rest period should be equal to, or slightly longer than, the surge period; this allows the muscle to relax fully, preventing muscle fatigue and build up of lactic acid which would cause pain. It should not be too long as this is a waste of time. Many modern machines have an inbuilt automatic optimum relaxation time.

4 **Ramp-time** This controls the rate of rise of the current; individual pulses are inhibited gradually to give build-up to peak flow. Sharp rises give the best response. The rate must not be too slow as the muscle will accommodate.

5 **Frequency control/pulses per second/Hz** This controls the number of pulses per second. The importance of frequency is discussed fully on page 181. Frequency determines the strength of contraction at the motor unit. Different fibre types will respond differently to different frequencies. Up to 20 Hz only the slow fibres will be showing smooth, fused tetanic contraction. At 40 Hz the majority of fibres will be showing fused tetanic contractions, although some fast fibres may require a higher frequency. Therefore, by selecting a frequency of 40 to 60 Hz, most fibres in the muscle will be contracting smoothly. The frequency within this range can be selected to provide the most

comfortable smooth contraction for the client. If there is a tremor in the muscle, a higher frequency is needed. There is nothing to be gained by selecting frequencies over 80 Hz as near maximal force is developed in human muscle with frequencies between 40 and 80 Hz. Some machines offer timed sequences beginning with lower frequencies moving through middle into higher frequencies.

6 **Phase control** This offers biphasic or monophasic pulses.

(a) *Monophasic/uniphasic/single pulses* The current flows mainly in one direction, therefore the polarity of the pads remains the same for each contraction. One will be $(-)$, the cathode, and the other $(+)$, the anode. Leads usually indicate this by one having a groove or being rounded – check with the manufacturer's instructions to establish which is which. As the cathode produces the greatest response, it should always be placed on the weaker muscle. This is useful for split and duplicate motor point padding if one muscle is weaker than another. If muscles are of equal power, and for longitudinal padding, biphasic pulses may be used.

(b) *Biphasic/dual pulses* The current behaves like AC as alternate pulses are reversed: it therefore eliminates polarity. It provides an even current under both pads.

7 **Mode control/programme control** This controls the rhythms of the contraction and relaxation times.

(a) *Constant* The rhythm of the programme remains the same once selected. The length of surge and interval remain the same throughout treatment.

(b) *Variable/rhythmic/active* The rhythm of the surge and interval vary throughout the treatment. This has the advantage of preventing the client anticipating the contraction and resisting it (useful with tense, nervous clients). In many modern machines, a selection of variable contraction times will give the muscles thorough non-repetitious exercise.

8 **Pulse width** This alters the width of each pulse; when the pulse width is increased, it has a similar effect to increasing the intensity control. This is because additional current is provided as the pulse is on for a longer period. Pulse widths under 100 μs are not effective; over 300 μs can be uncomfortable. A medium width of between 200 and 300 μs produces a good contraction. Select 150–200 μs at the commencement of treatment, and if the client cannot tolerate an increase in intensity due to discomfort, increase the pulse width, which may produce a better contraction.

9 **Maximum and minimum gain/master output** This control increases the current to all the outlets being used – to increase the intensity when the client has got

used to the sensation. This control can be at zero at commencement of treatment, or it can be set midway so that the intensity can be increased or decreased during treatment.

10 **Intensity controls (output controls) and pulse amplitude** These control the current flowing through each pair of pads. Most machines have an intensity control for one pair of pads; however, there are machines where two pairs of pads share the same intensity control.

> The intensity is increased to produce a good visible contraction but it must be within the tolerance of the client.

As the intensity control is turned up, the amount of current flowing through the pad increases. When selecting intensity, 'a good visible contraction within the tolerance of the client' is the best guide. Avoid turning the intensity too high, thinking that a stronger contraction is always better. Muscle fibres obey the 'all or none law', that is once the stimulus is great enough to produce a contraction, there will be no increase in response by turning up the intensity. However, as the intensity of the current is increased, the strength of contraction is seen to increase. This is because more motor units are stimulated. Some machines have numbers around the intensity control which serve as a rough guide. The intensity control will be turned up to obtain optimum maximum contraction with minimum discomfort.

The Placement of Pads (Electrodes)

The correct placement of pads is very important and will affect the outcome of the treatment. In order to pad effectively, the therapist must understand the methods of padding and must know the position of the motor points of the superficial muscles. A pad placed anywhere on the muscle will initiate a response, but may well be uncomfortable. The most effective and comfortable contraction is obtained if a muscle is stimulated at the motor point, that is where the nerve enters the muscle belly (see page 178). Motor point padding should always be used if possible, as it allows very precise targeting of muscles and enables suitable intensities to be selected for individual muscles. Stimulation here is more effective at

lower intensities and is therefore more comfortable for the client. Bilateral padding is usually used in beauty therapy as improvement is required on both sides of the body. Various names are given to varieties of padding.

Longitudinal padding

In the past, this method used the pads near the origin and insertion of the muscle. However, as muscle function may be impaired by padding off the motor points, longitudinal padding must now mean padding on the upper and lower motor points of a muscle. This is only possible on long muscles with more than one motor point. This is an excellent method of motor point padding as all the current is applied to one muscle and the intensity is controlled to gain maximum contraction of the muscle. Also as the current from one pair of pads is applied to one muscle, a lower intensity will produce the desired contraction, which will be more comfortable for the client. This would always be the method of choice for muscles with two motor points. The next pair of pads is applied to the same muscle on the other side of the body. Muscles which may be padded longitudinally include: rectus abdominis, rectus femoris, gracilis, trapezius, triceps.

Duplicate padding

A pair of pads is placed on the motor points of two adjacent muscles; the next pair is placed on the same two muscles on the other side of the body. This method has the disadvantage that the intensity cannot be controlled to individual muscles, and muscles may require different intensities if one is weaker than another. The use of monophasic pulses will help if the cathode is placed on the weaker muscle. As the current is divided, a higher intensity may be required to produce the desired contraction and will be less comfortable for the client. When using duplicate motor point padding, always try to pad muscles with the same or similar action.

Muscles which are suitable for duplicate padding include: gluteus medius and tensor fasciae latae (abductors); adductor longus and gracilis (adductors); external oblique and rectus abdominis (abdominals).

Split padding

One pair of pads is split and placed on the motor point of the same muscle, but on opposite sides of the body. Again the current is divided between two muscles, which prevents individual control. If one side of the body is weaker than the other, monophasic pulses should be used and the cathode placed on the weaker muscle. If muscles are of equal strength, biphasic pulses should be used. This is a useful method for using up the last pair of pads. Muscles suitable for split padding include: right and left pectorals; right and left triceps; right and left gluteus maximus.

Factors to be borne in mind when padding

1 Always pad on motor points if possible.

2 Use longitudinal padding if a muscle has more than one motor point. The intensity can be selected to obtain maximum contraction of that muscle.

3 For optimum contraction, place a muscle in its relaxed mid range position.

4 The brain does not register individual muscle movement, but rather patterns of movement. During normal body movement, antagonistic muscles do not contract together. When the prime mover contracts, the antagonist relaxes. Therefore, when simulating movement, the padding of opposite muscles should be avoided. In practice it is not always possible to adhere rigidly to this rule, and providing there is no movement at the joint, opposing muscles are sometimes padded (e.g. the adductors and abductors of the hip joint).

Some units are designed to stimulate antagonistic muscles alternately; this would seem a good idea.

When using duplicate padding, do not use one pair on antagonistic muscles as one is likely to be weaker than the other and the intensity to each group cannot be individually controlled.

5 Consider the phase control when padding. With biphasic current the contractions are even under both pads. With monophasic current the cathode is stronger and should therefore be used where one muscle of a pair may be weaker than the other (very useful for duplicate and split padding).

Methods of padding should be selected and adapted to suit the needs of individual clients. Having decided on padding methods, other factors should be considered which will influence the response:

1 Thoroughly cleansing the skin to remove sebum and dirt (wash with warm soapy water or use cologne).

2 Pre-heating the muscles with some form of heat treatment will increase the response, for example infra-red, sauna, or steam bath (which is particularly effective as it also moistens the skin).

3 Ensuring the accurate positioning of electrodes/pads on the motor points.

4 Selecting appropriate control settings.

REMEMBER! Fat impedes the flow of current, and the treatment will be ineffective if the muscles are covered by a deep layer of fat. Muscle stimulation is also ineffective on deep muscles. Padding should be selected for superficial muscles only.

Factors governing the strength of the contractions

Many factors influence the strength of contractions. Output controls regulate the amount of current flowing to the tissues, but are little guide to the amount of contraction. The strength of contraction varies and depends on many factors:

1 The size of the muscle and the selection of appropriate padding.

2 The number of motor units activated.

3 The depth of the muscle – EMS is effective on superficial muscles only.

4 The amount of covering fat – fat is an insulator; therefore, current will not pass through very fatty areas.

5 The condition of the muscle – well-toned muscles respond to lower intensity of current.

6 The rate of rise of the current – a sharp rise produces a contraction, a slow rise allows for accommodation of the muscle fibres.

7 Moist skin offers less resistance to the current.

8 Warm muscles contract more readily.

9 Firm, even padding giving good surface contact will ensure maximum effect.

Motor Points of the Superficial Body Muscles

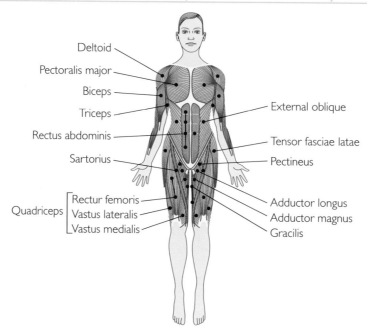

Deltoid
Pectoralis major
Biceps
Triceps
Rectus abdominis
Sartorius
Quadriceps { Rectur femoris
Vastus lateralis
Vastus medialis

External oblique
Tensor fasciae latae
Pectineus
Adductor longus
Adductor magnus
Gracilis

Figure 9.20   Superficial muscles and motor points (anterior)

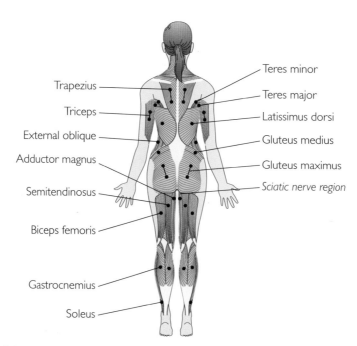

Trapezius
Triceps
External oblique
Adductor magnus
Semitendinosus
Biceps femoris
Gastrocnemius
Soleus

Teres minor
Teres major
Latissimus dorsi
Gluteus medius
Gluteus maximus
Sciatic nerve region

Figure 9.21   Superficial muscles and motor points (posterior)

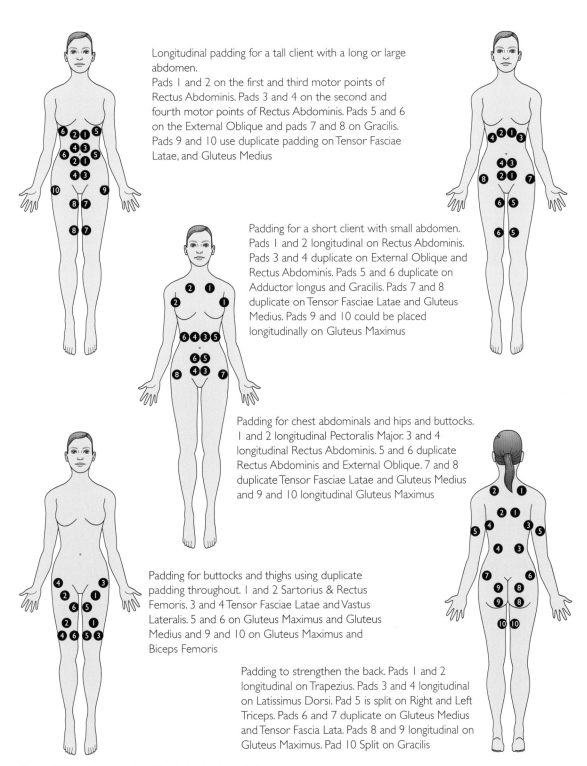

Longitudinal padding for a tall client with a long or large abdomen.
Pads 1 and 2 on the first and third motor points of Rectus Abdominis. Pads 3 and 4 on the second and fourth motor points of Rectus Abdominis. Pads 5 and 6 on the External Oblique and pads 7 and 8 on Gracilis. Pads 9 and 10 use duplicate padding on Tensor Fasciae Latae, and Gluteus Medius

Padding for a short client with small abdomen.
Pads 1 and 2 longitudinal on Rectus Abdominis. Pads 3 and 4 duplicate on External Oblique and Rectus Abdominis. Pads 5 and 6 duplicate on Adductor longus and Gracilis. Pads 7 and 8 duplicate on Tensor Fasciae Latae and Gluteus Medius. Pads 9 and 10 could be placed longitudinally on Gluteus Maximus

Padding for chest abdominals and hips and buttocks.
1 and 2 longitudinal Pectoralis Major. 3 and 4 longitudinal Rectus Abdominis. 5 and 6 duplicate Rectus Abdominis and External Oblique. 7 and 8 duplicate Tensor Fasciae Latae and Gluteus Medius and 9 and 10 longitudinal Gluteus Maximus

Padding for buttocks and thighs using duplicate padding throughout. 1 and 2 Sartorius & Rectus Femoris. 3 and 4 Tensor Fasciae Latae and Vastus Lateralis. 5 and 6 on Gluteus Maximus and Gluteus Medius and 9 and 10 on Gluteus Maximus and Biceps Femoris

Padding to strengthen the back. Pads 1 and 2 longitudinal on Trapezius. Pads 3 and 4 longitudinal on Latissimus Dorsi. Pad 5 is split on Right and Left Triceps. Pads 6 and 7 duplicate on Gluteus Medius and Tensor Fascia Lata. Pads 8 and 9 longitudinal on Gluteus Maximus. Pad 10 Split on Gracilis

Figure 9.22   Suggested methods for body padding

Uses

1 Figure reshaping, particularly when used in conjunction with active exercise.

2 To re-educate muscles with poor tone due to prolonged disuse (e.g. adductors and triceps).

3 To restore muscle tone of abdominals after pregnancy.

4 To firm the pectoral muscles, which may correct breast sag.

5 To firm body contours and maintain an attractive figure, while losing body weight through dieting.

> EMS is effective on superficial muscles only. It will not penetrate the deeper layers nor a covering of fat.

Effects

1 The stimulation of motor nerves resulting in muscle contraction. The selection of an appropriate frequency will produce contraction of most fibres of a muscle. (This differs from active movement when only a percentage of fibres contract: it therefore improves muscle tone.)

2 It improves the circulation due to the pumping action of the contracting muscles. This increases the nutrients and oxygen brought to the body part and speeds up the removal of waste products.

3 It increases the metabolic rate, which improves the condition of the muscle.

4 It stimulates the sensory nerve, giving the prickling sensation.

5 It produces vasodilation and erythema under the pads.

> EMS will restore muscle tone but will not strengthen muscles. Resisted exercises must be given to improve muscle strength.

Contraindications

1 Muscle injury or spasm.

2 Broken bones.

3 Extensive cuts and bruises (small cuts may be insulated with petroleum jelly).

4 Skin disorders and diseases.

5 Recent scar tissue.

6 Metal pins and plates (superficial).

7 Pacemakers.

8 Heart conditions.

9 High or low blood pressure.

10 Thrombosis.

11 Phlebitis.

Dangers

■ There are no specific dangers to EMS. Discomfort can be caused if the intensity is too high, if the pads are in the wrong position, that is not on motor points, over bony points or over any open abrasions that are not insulated.

- Muscle fatigue can be produced if the intensity is too high, the rest interval is too short or the treatment is prolonged.
- Heavy padding of the chest region should be avoided as stimuli may interfere with heart rhythm.

Precautions

1 When the intensity is turned up, *never* move the pads, press pads down or push the terminals in.

2 Check for contraindications.

3 Test the machine.

4 Select appropriate points on all controls.

5 Ensure the intensity controls are at zero.

6 Check the pads and wet them with saline or water.

7 Strap the pads securely.

8 Check the outlets before switching the machine on.

9 Turn *up* during the *surge* only, the client must be able to feel the current increasing and tell you if it becomes uncomfortable.

10 Turn down and switch off during the rest period.

11 Avoid heavy padding of chest region: pad anterior or posterior but not both.

Treatment technique

Preparation of the client

1 Position the client in a comfortable, well-supported position.

2 Remove jewellery.

3 Check for contraindications.

4 Pre-heat the body using steam, sauna, infra-red/radiant heat or shower – heat improves muscle action and moistens the skin, thus lowering its resistance.

5 Explain the treatment to the client, that is a prickling sensation followed by contraction; reassure the client and encourage her to relax.

> Turn the intensity to zero before performing any of the following
>
> - moving the pads
> - applying pressure to the pads
> - pushing the terminals into the socket.

Procedure

1 Place the machine on a suitable stable base and check that the plugs and leads are secure.

2 Check that the intensity controls are at zero.

3 Collect all commodities, hot water or saline solution, cotton wool, talc, cologne and a selection of straps of varying lengths.

4 Check the machine on yourself.

5　Check skin for cuts, abrasions and insulate them with petroleum jelly or cover with plaster. If the client has not taken a shower, clean the skin by washing or wiping with cologne or surgical spirit.

6　Select a suitable padding layout and make a note of it on a record card.

7　Secure the straps around the body.

8　Moisten the surfaces of the pads evenly and place them accurately over the identified motor points; ensure a firm even contact.

9　Select the appropriate controls, frequency, mode, etc.

10　Check that the intensity controls are at zero.

11　Switch the machine on and turn each intensity control up slowly until a good visible contraction is obtained.

12　Cover the client and keep her warm.

13　As the client grows accustomed to the sensation, and as pads dry out slightly, the intensity may be increased after a few minutes.

14　The treatment should end after 30–40 minutes. Switch off.

15　Turn all dials to zero.

16　Remove the pads in reverse order to avoid tangling.

17　Dry and talc treated area.

18　Clean the pads with warm water and detergent.

19　The treatment can be carried out two to three times per week for six to eight weeks as required.

20　The client should be taught exercises to carry out at home to increase the effectiveness of the treatment.

REMEMBER! Feedback and after care.

Do not position the pads over bony points or too near muscle tendons.

Reasons for poor contractions

1　The intensity is too low.

2　The pads are too dry or dirty.

3　There is grease on the skin.

4　Treating over a depth of fat.

5　Incorrect positioning of pads, off motor points or near tendons. (Motor points are never found near tendons.)

6　Poor contact between the pads and skin. Avoid bony points as it is difficult to obtain even contact, the current will concentrate at the bony point.

7　Poor contact at leads and loose terminals.

Patterns of padding for use on the body

In order to pad accurately, therapists must understand the three methods of padding and the position of the motor points of the superficial body muscles. Padding should then be selected to suit the client. Some suggestions are shown in Figure 9.22 on page 199.

Check list

Have you carried out the following points of technique?

- Conducted a client consultation.
- Discussed the treatment with the client.
- Checked for contraindications.
- Removed all jewellery.
- Carried out a skin sensitivity test.
- Offered a suitable form of pre-heating treatment. Warm muscles contract more readily than cold muscles and moist skin offers less resistance to the current. A lower intensity of current will thus produce a good contraction, which will be more comfortable for the client.
- Prepared the machine and all the commodities in accordance with safety requirements.
- Placed the client in a comfortable, warm, relaxed position.
- Explained the treatment and the prickling sensation to the client.
- Cleaned the area with surgical spirit to ensure that all sebum or dirt is removed as these are a barrier to the current.
- Examined the area for any cuts or abrasions and covered these with water proof plaster.
- Selected the most appropriate method of padding to suit the client and the desired outcomes.
- Identified the motor points of the selected muscles.
- Identified all the controls on the machine and ensured that you know the effects when adjusting each control.
- Tested the current on yourself.

- Placed the strapping in position.
- Moistened the covers evenly, squeezing out excess saline.
- Positioned the pads under the straps ensuring firm, even pressure leaving no air gaps.
- Checked that the plug, leads, etc. are sound and secure.
- Checked that all the terminals and controls are accurately located and secure.
- Checked that all the controls are at zero before switching the machine on.
- Selected the appropriate output at each control.
- Ensured that the rest period is the same as or slightly longer than the contraction time to prevent muscle fatigue.
- Turned the intensity control up slowly during the surge and turned down during rest period.
- Ensured the best visible contraction within the tolerance of the client.
- Covered the client and ensured her comfort and warmth.
- Remained within calling distance of the client throughout the treatment.
- Ensured that the intensity controls were at zero before making any adjustments to the pads i.e. moving or applying pressure to the pads or pushing the terminals into the sockets.
- Treatment time 30–40 minutes.
- Removed pads in reverse order.
- Dried the area and applied talc.
- Washed the pads with warm water and detergent.

Therapists need to remember that the long or large abdomen requires more pads than the small abdomen so use the four motor points of rectus abdominis and pad external oblique longitudinally. The internal oblique and transverus abdominis are too deep for stimulation. For the abductor muscles, tensor fasciae latae, gluteus medius and the deep minimus which give shape to the thigh, insert high up on the thigh. Gluteus medius and the deep minimus both insert into the greater trochanter of the femur, but tensor fasciae latae inserts into the lateral fascia of the thigh. Therefore padding on the top and bottom of the outside of the thigh will not target these muscles. This method of padding will target tensor fasciae latae and vastus lateralis.

In the past beauty therapists have avoided padding the quadriceps group as their strength is maintained through constant use. However, there is now a growing desire among some members of the general public for athletic looking legs and quadriceps can be padded to achieve this aim. The quadriceps muscles could be padded as follows: rectus femoris may be duplicated with sartorius, vastus medialis may be duplicated with gracilis, vastus lateralis may be duplicated with tensor fasciae latae. Vastus intermedius is too deep for stimulation.

Triceps may be padded longitudinally or split. This will improve the tone at the posterior aspect of the upper arm. Biceps rarely needs improvement in tone as it is in constant use. Do not stimulate biceps and triceps together as contraction of these muscles will move the elbow joint.

Placing the client in a low half-lying position will achieve better abdominal contractions as the muscles are relaxed and will contract in mid range.

SUMMARY

- Electrical impulses produced by machines will stimulate motor nerves resulting in the contraction of muscles supplied by those nerves.
- Muscles are composed of bundles of muscle fibres.
- Motor nerves (or neurones) transmit impulses from the brain and spinal cord to the muscle fibres.
- The **motor end plate** is the modification of the muscle fibre at the point where the nerve terminal comes close to it. The synapse between the end of the nerve and the muscle fibre it supplies is known as the **neuro-muscular junction.**
- The **motor point** is the point where the motor nerve enters the belly of the muscle; after entering the muscle it divides into many branches. Each branch supplies a single muscle fibre.
- The **motor unit** includes the anterior horn cell, its axon, axon branches and all the muscle fibres supplied by that axon.

summary continues overleaf

summary continued from previous page

- One motor unit will supply hundreds of muscle fibres, therefore, many motor units are required to supply a whole muscle.

- Each muscle is made up of different types of muscle fibre, that is slow oxidative fibres, fast oxidative glycolytic fibres and fast glycolytic fibres.

- These fibres respond in different ways to different rates of frequencies of impulses: slow fibres contract smoothly (tetanically) to low frequencies up to 20 Hz; fast fibres contract smoothly (tetanically) to higher frequencies up to 80 Hz.

- Smooth, tetanic muscle contraction is obtained at frequencies of between 40–80 Hz.

Electrical stimulation

- Pulses must be of sufficient duration and intensity to produce a contraction (high frequency currents have pulses of short duration and will not stimulate motor nerves).

- A sharply rising pulse produces the best contraction; slow rising pulses allow the muscle to accommodate. Pulses are grouped together in trains or envelopes with rest periods in between.

- When the current flows, the muscles contract; when the current stops, the muscles relax.

- Pulses are surged so that each pulse increases in intensity to peak value and then decreases. The rate of rise of the current is known as the ramp time. The frequency of the current is the number of pulses per second. Different muscle fibres respond differently to different frequencies. Only slow fibres will contract smoothly/tetanically to frequencies under 20 Hz, the fast fibres require frequencies of around 60–80 Hz to produce smooth tetanic contractions.

- Frequencies in the range 40–80 Hz will produce good tetanic contractions when using EMS. A few minutes at the lower range of 20 Hz, moving into middle range 40–60 Hz and then to 80 Hz and back to middle gives a thorough treatment.

- The intensity selected should produce 'a good visible contraction' within the tolerance of the client.

Phasic controls

- Monophasic selection means that one pad is slightly stronger than the other; the cathode is stronger than the anode. This may be used for duplicate or split padding if one muscle is weaker than the other when the cathode would be used on the weaker muscle.

- Biphasic selection means that alternate pulses are reversed, which eliminates polarity; the current is even under both pads. This may be used with longitudinal padding or with other methods if the muscles are of equal strength.

- The pulse width selected is between 200 and 300 μs.

summary continues overleaf

summary continued from previous page

- Always use motor point padding.
- There are three methods used on the body:
  1. Longitudinal: a pair of pads are on one muscle, one on the upper motor point, the other on the lower motor point. Repeat this on the other side of the body.
  2. Duplicate: a pair of pads are on two adjacent muscles, one on the motor point of one muscle, the other on the motor point of the other muscle. Repeat this on the other side of the body.
  3. Split padding: a pair of pads are on the same muscle, but on opposite sides of the body, one on the motor point of the right muscle, the other on the motor point of the left muscle.
- There are two methods commonly used on the face:
  1. Facial disc electrode: a disc is used as the active electrode and is used over the motor point of individual muscles. The inactive electrode is strapped on to the arm or behind the shoulder.
  2. Facial inactive and active combined electrode: this contains both electrodes, and is placed over the branches of the facial nerve to stimulate many muscles simultaneously.

Questions

1. Describe the composition of skeletal muscle.
2. List the parts of the nervous system.
3. Define the following:
   (a) motor point
   (b) neuro-muscular junction
   (c) motor end plate
   (d) motor unit.
4. List three types of muscle fibres and give the transmission frequencies to produce smooth contractions of each fibre type.
5. Why should the electrodes/pads be placed on the motor point of a muscle?
6. Give three uses for electrical muscle stimulation of the face.
7. Explain three methods used for padding superficial body muscles.
8. Explain the difference in muscle response when using a disc electrode or a combined facial electrode when stimulating facial muscles.
9. Explain the purpose of the following controls found on machines:
   (a) intensity control
   (b) surge length

questions continues overleaf

questions continued from previous page

    (c) relaxation length
    (d) phasic control
    (e) pulse width
    (f) maximum/minimum gain or master control
    (g) rhythm control.

10   The intensity of current is one factor that governs the strength of contractions; list six other factors which determine the strength of contractions.

11   List six contraindications to each of the following:
    (a) Stimulation of facial muscles.
    (b) Stimulation of body muscles.

12   Give three uses for electrical muscle stimulation of body muscles.

13   Give the dangers of electrical stimulation of body muscles.

14   Describe four factors which may result in poor contractions.

Oral questions

Facial electrical muscle stimulation (facial faradic)

1   What type of current is used to stimulate facial muscles?
2   When would the use of muscle stimulation be indicated?
3   How is the current applied to the client?
4   When using the disc electrode where would you place it and why?
5   What is meant by the motor point?
6   When using the block electrode where would you place it?
7   Are there disadvantages in using the facial mask?
8   (a) Which muscle(s) would you work on if the client had a double chin?
    (b) Which muscle produces horizontal wrinkles over the bridge of the nose?
    (c) What is the action of masseter?
9   Are there any specific safety factors which you must consider with this treatment?
10   How many contractions would you give each muscle?
11   How long is the treatment?

Body electrical muscle stimulation (body faradic)

1   What type of current is used?
2   How is the current applied to the client?
3   Why would you suggest EMS for a client?
4   Where should the pads be placed?
5   How many ways/methods of padding are there?

questions continues overleaf

questions continued from previous page

6   Explain the method of padding you would use for long muscles.

7   Name the method of padding where a pair of pads are placed on adjacent muscles with similar action and repeated on the other side of the body.

8   What is the main disadvantage of split padding?

9   If the contractions were poor what action would you take?

10   How would you prevent muscle fatigue?

11   Are there any other dangers?

12   Why must you cover open wounds with petroleum jelly and a waterproof plaster?

13   What treatment would you suggest prior to EMS? Give reasons why.

14   What is the benefit of heating tissue?

15   How long would the treatment last?

16   Complete the following chart:

Machine controls	Function	Special points
On/off switch	_____	Make sure all terminals are at zero
Surge control/ surge envelope	_____	Muscles with poor tone require a _____ surge
Relaxation control/ rest period	Controls the length of rest period	Must be _____ than the surge
Frequency control	Controls the number of _____ per second	Should be set between _____

Microcurrent Treatment

Microcurrent is very low intensity, direct current which is modified to produce low frequency pulses of differing wave forms. The current is delivered in microamps (μA), which is of lower intensity than the previous direct current used in galvanic treatments and the modified/pulsed direct current used in muscle stimulating treatments which was delivered in milliamps (mA). One milliamp equals one thousand microamps.

Microcurrent therapy has been used in the medical field for many years to promote tissue healing: these very low intensity electrical currents stimulate the cells' metabolic processes. Microcurrents are more closely related to the body's own bio-electrical activity and augment the body's own healing process. Research indicates that weak stimuli increase physiological activity whereas very strong stimuli inhibit, therefore these small pulses of current are more effective and beneficial in improving the condition of the tissues than the previously used stronger stimuli.

Microcurrent is used in beauty therapy to maintain a youthful appearance and combat the effects of ageing on the skin. The current increases the circulation of blood and lymph; accelerates intracellular processes and the exchange of substances across cell membranes; improves the metabolic rate and is thought to normalize the activity within the cells; stimulates myofibrils thus improving muscle function; and in addition it can be used for its polar effects under the cathode or anode depending on the electrode connections (in the same way as the galvanic treatments).

Figure 9.23   A microcurrent unit for facial and body treatment

Being of low intensity, the current is not as irritating to sensory nerves. It produces lower grade sensations and is therefore less painful for the client and can be tolerated for a longer time. It is safe to use because the machines are usually battery powered and not connected to the mains which eliminates the danger of mains electric shock. However if the machine is mains operated, then the transformer is used to step down the voltage and isolate the output which also eliminates the danger of mains shock.

These treatments are becoming very popular as they are effective and feel more comfortable than those previously available. They are well advertised by the manufacturers and clients are aware of their effects, uses and advantages. Demand is increasing and more and more salons are offering these treatments. At the present time they are predominantly advertised as a facial lifting treatment but many systems include programmes for body treatment.

Machines

Microcurrent units/machines/systems produce direct current of very low amperage which is modified to produce low frequency pulses of current with different wave forms.

As stated above, most of the older type direct current machines used for galvanic treatments or modified for muscle stimulation treatments delivered current flow in milliamps. Microcurrent machines deliver current flow in microamps.

1 milliamp = 1/1000 of an amp

1 microamp = 1/1000 of a milliamp

Microcurrent units for the beauty market vary widely in design and cost: they start at around two hundred pounds and go up to five or six thousand pounds. Basically they all use the latest electronic microchip technology to produce similar small pulses of current but they differ in their design, modalities and in the number and type of programmes offered. Most of the units/ systems available offer multiple preset programmes for different conditions and different areas of the face and body.

The direct current is used for disincrustation and iontophoresis. Other treatments are possible because electronic devices in the machine modify the direct current. The flow is made to start and stop at regular intervals; to rise sharply or gradually, producing a selection of wave forms of different duration and frequency.

Examples of wave forms:

- sine wave
- square or rectangular wave
- triangular
- trapezoidal
- saw tooth or ramp

Sine wave/alternating wave form

Alternating current has no polarity and will not produce muscle contraction; it is used for its stimulating effects on metabolism, blood circulation and lymphatic drainage. Some machines have an auto build-up setting where the intensity varies within each cycle from minimum to maximum values.

Interrupted/pulsed direct current

The type of pulses offered on the machine will vary: some systems offer a wider variety than others. They may be preprogrammed or a wave form control may be available, allowing selection. The indications for use will be explained in the instruction manual for your machine.

As explained earlier, interrupted direct current can be used to stimulate motor nerves which will result in a contraction of the muscles supplied by that nerve. However if the current intensity is insufficient to stimulate the motor nerves, a muscle contraction may still be produced through direct stimulation of the muscle fibres. Microcurrent is low intensity current, too low to stimulate the motor nerves, but providing the intensity of the current and the duration of the impulses are adequate, the muscle fibres will be stimulated directly and will contract. The contraction will be weaker and not as visible as the contraction produced by the nerve stimulating higher amperage faradic-type currents. With microcurrent treatment there is no visible contraction of the muscle. However some systems are designed to produce adequate higher intensity pulses which will stimulate the muscle fibres in this way.

Research indicates that when an adequate interrupted current is applied to a muscle, a contraction of the fibres and shortening of the muscle will result. However, claims are made that microcurrent will stimulate the sensory receptors within the muscles and their tendons. These include **muscle spindles** which control the degree of stretch and **Golgi organs** which affect the degree of tension within the muscle. By adapting the technique of application, microcurrent may be effective in tightening slack muscles *and* stretching tight muscles. The author can find no scientific research evidence to support these claims and the way in which these two opposite functions can be achieved is unclear.

However the beneficial physiological changes that occur in the muscle will

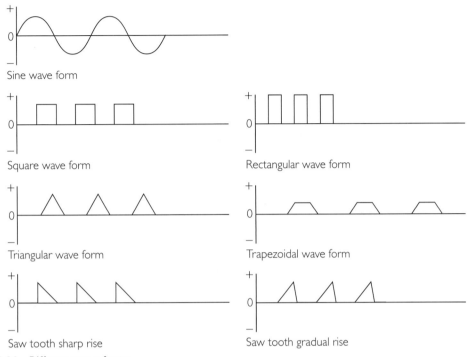

Figure 9.24   Different wave forms

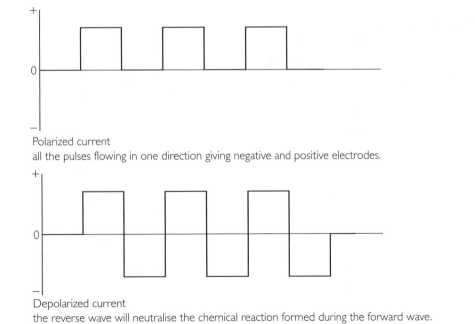

Polarized current
all the pulses flowing in one direction giving negative and positive electrodes.

Depolarized current
the reverse wave will neutralise the chemical reaction formed during the forward wave.

Figure 9.25   Polarized and depolarized current

improve its condition and function but will not increase strength.

A course of 10–12 treatments over a period of time is required to bring about this improvement. Visual observation of facial contours before and after treatment will indicate improvement.

Although pulsed, the current will be polarized as each pulse is flowing in the same direction and will produce galvanic effects. One electrode will be positive and the other negative depending on the electrode connections and as with galvanic current, chemical changes/reactions will take place under the electrodes. This current can therefore be used for its chemical polar effects and to repel beneficial ionized preparations into the skin (iontophoresis). It is also used by some systems for the moisturising phase of the programme.

When the effects at the cathode are required, the negative electrode must be the working (active) electrode, the other electrode, the anode, must be stationary and away from the area. When the effects at the anode are required, the positive electrode must be the active electrode and the cathode will be stationary and away from the area.

If this polar effect is not required, some systems reverse the current between impulses to give depolarized current. The chemicals produced at the poles during the forward impulse are neutralized by the reverse wave.

Controls

These will vary depending on which machine you are using. The instruction manual will explain the function of each control and their mode of action. If you are in doubt ask the manufacturer.

Examples of machine controls

- On/off switch/button: this switches on the power to the unit.

- Intensity switch/button/dial: this increases or decreases the current flow. Some units have a dial which is turned up to increase the amount of current flowing and turned down to decrease the current. Other systems have buttons for selecting low, medium, high. The intensity selected will depend on the area being treated and the tolerance of the client.

  Microcurrent treatments should always be comfortable: a very, very mild tingling sensation should be felt. Some areas such as around the eyes will be more sensitive than others and will require lower intensity. Current values can vary from around $10\,\mu A$ up to around $600\,\mu A$ and even higher up to and above $1\,000\,\mu A$ into the milli-amp range.

- Wave form: most units produce a selection of wave forms as explained above. The method in which they generate these may differ but the effects they produce will be similar. The training manual will indicate selection.

- Frequency: some machines allow selection of frequency, that is the number of pulses per second, but this is usually pre-programmed.

- Polarity switch/button: this allows selection of negative or positive electrode (depending on the electrode connections). Selection will depend on whether the effects under the cathode or anode are required.

- Programme selector: this allows the programme to be selected depending on the effect required and the part of the body being treated. Different machines offer different pre-set programmes, so read the instruction manual thoroughly to ensure that you select the most suitable for the client.

- Timer: this allows the time to be set for each area. A tone, bell or buzzer will sound when the treatment of each area is complete.

    Timing is important when giving microcurrent treatments as some areas will require a longer time than others but equal timing *must* be given to each side of the face or body to ensure an even result.

Application of current

The current may be applied manually using probe or roller electrodes or may be applied automatically using small adhesive electrodes placed on appropriate points on the skin. Most of the systems are designed for use by a trained therapist but a few of the simple to operate pre-programmed units are on sale to the general public.

    Before purchasing a system make sure that you thoroughly investigate the market. Look at as many systems as possible, ask for a demonstration, read the training manual thoroughly and you can then make an informed choice and select the most suitable unit to meet your needs. *You must then receive product training from the manufacturer.* This is essential because the treatment procedure will be specific to the system you choose. Systems vary widely in design, the number and type of programmes offered, the terminology

used and the complexity of operation. You must always closely follow the instruction manual which accompanies your particular machine.

Types of electrodes

The current is delivered to the client by means of two or more electrodes. The current flows from one, through the skin, to the other, the client completing the circuit. The electrodes vary in design depending on the system.

Small adhesive electrodes

These are small round or square electrodes that are attached to leads which have terminal connections to the machine. They have a conductive adhesive side and a non-conductive rubberized side. They are applied to the skin at specific points to provide automatic treatment. This method of application frees the therapist to do other things. The pattern of application depends on the required effect; follow the diagrams in the instruction manual.

Rollers

These are small metal rollers which move easily over the surface of the skin and are attached to handles with a terminal lead connection. The recommended product must be spread evenly over the face and the rollers moved slowly and evenly over the entire area. Always keep a space between the rollers when working; if the rollers touch, the current will flow from one to another and not through the client's skin. For body work many rollers may be grouped together to form a block which covers a large area, such as the back, more efficiently.

Probes

These are long pencil-like electrodes with a lead connection to one end and a metal head or socket on the other. Cotton wool or cotton buds are inserted into these sockets. Some probes have only one socket for one cotton bud while others have two sockets for two cotton buds (i.e. twin buds in each electrode). This gives greater coverage.

Probes are used in pairs, the current flowing from one to the other through the tissues. They may be moved at the same time, either towards or away from each other, or one may be held stationary while the other moves away or towards it.

Some units have both electrodes in one holder making it easier to use. Both electrodes must be in contact with the skin for the current flow. The skin and probes must be kept moist throughout, usually with water and a specific anti-ageing preparation supplied by the manufacturer.

Gloves

Some systems have gloves which are attached to leads. The therapist wears the gloves and moves her hands over the moistened part in massage-type movements. This is a good way of covering large areas.

Other ways of delivering the current are continually being developed.

Effects

General effects

- Increases the circulation to the skin, bringing more oxygen and nutrients to the cells and speeding up the removal of metabolites (waste products).
- Improves lymphatic drainage thus reducing puffiness.
- Improves the permeability of the cell membrane, allowing easier passage of substances in and out of the cells.
- Increases cell metabolism which will improve the condition of the skin.
- Increases the production of ATP (adenosine triphosphate), the break-down of which provides the energy for cellular activity.
- Improves protein synthesis which improves the condition of the tissues.
- Stimulates activity of the basal layer and cell mitosis which enhances skin renewal.
- Improves ion exchange which normalizes the activity of deficient cells and aids the repair of damaged cells thus augmenting the body's own healing processes.
- Stimulates the fibroblasts which improve the production of collagen and elastin.
- Stimulates myofibrils, improving muscle condition and function. It is claimed that by adapting the technique, a slack, atrophied muscle can be toned and shortened, or a tight muscle can be stretched, but the mode in which this is achieved is unclear.
- Low intensity current and good technique may produce a general relaxing effect.

Effects when the cathode is used as the active electrode

- The alkali, sodium hydroxide, will saponify sebum and soften the skin. This will have a deep cleansing effect. It will also break down keratin in the superficial layers of the skin, aiding desquamation.

- Water is drawn towards the cathode which produces a temporary hydrating effect, this softens the skin and any scar tissue.

- Produces vasodilation with hyperaemia and erythema.

- Increases conductivity and excitability of nerves.

- Hydrogen is released, improving the vitality of the tissues.

- Products containing negatively charged ions will be repelled into the skin.

Effects when the anode is used as the active electrode

- The hydrochloric acid formed tightens and hardens the skin and has an astringent effect.

- Water moves away from the anode.

- Vasodilation with hyperaemia and erythema but not as great as under the cathode.

- Decreases the conductivity and excitability of nerves.

- Oxygen is released which will improve cell metabolism.

- Products containing positively charged ions will be repelled into the skin.

Uses

- To maintain a youthful appearance.

- To improve the condition of the ageing skin.

- To soften lines and wrinkles.

- To improve the colour and texture of the skin and promote a healthy glow.

- To improve muscle condition and function. It is claimed that by adapting the technique, lax muscles may be toned and shortened or tight muscles stretched.

- To improve the contours of the face.

- To reduce puffiness.

- To soften scar tissue.

- To reduce pain, tension and promote relaxation.

Contraindications

- Individuals with a cardiac pacemaker.

- Epilepsy.

- Avoid passing the current through the eyeball or cardiac area. When treating the eye region keep over the bone around the eye, do not pass across the eyeball.

- Malignant tumours or any undiagnosed growths or lumps.

- Avoid areas of recent bruising or any bleeding.

- On the body during pregnancy.

Precautions

There are no specific dangers with these treatments as most units are battery driven and the current values are very low. However there are some precautions to bear in mind:

- Check for contraindications.

- Check that all jewellery, contact lenses or hearing aids have been removed.

- Cleanse and tone the area thoroughly, removing all grease.

- Use only the cotton buds recommended by the manufacturer, some buds with plastic holders will be non-conductors of electricity.

- Wet the electrodes thoroughly and keep moist throughout the treatment.

- Apply the gel or lotion liberally according to the manufacturer's instructions.

- Follow the manufacturer's instructions carefully; always make sure that they are specific to the system that you are using.

- Use firm even pressure except around the eyes where pressure should be lighter.

- Move the probes slowly in a gliding action across the skin, 4–6 seconds per stroke.

- Keep to the correct timings and ensure that you give equal treatment to both sides of the face otherwise you will have an uneven result.

- Check that the client is comfortable and happy throughout the treatment.

Treatment and technique

Preparation of the client

- Place the client in a well-supported and comfortable position.

- Check that all jewellery, contact lenses, hearing aid have been removed.

- Check for contraindications.

- Explain the treatment and tell the client what to expect.

- Cleanse and tone the skin.

- Moisten the skin thoroughly with water or recommended product according to the manufacturer's instruction.

Procedure

- Position the machine on a stable base and check that the plugs, leads and terminals are secure.

- Select the appropriate controls.

- Check that the intensity is at zero.

- Select the electrodes, prepare them as instructed in the manual and secure them into the machine.

- Check that you have selected the correct polarity, if this is required for the treatment.

- Some units may be tested by touching the electrodes, switching on and turning up the intensity; a signal will indicate that the current is flowing.

- Moisten the area and the electrodes thoroughly according to the manufacturer's instructions.

Figure 9.26   Examples of treatment

You are now ready to perform the treatment. The technique will be specific to the effect required and to the system you are using. Although there are some similarities, it is not possible to cover all the variations in this book. You must carefully adhere to the instructions issued by the manufacturer as these will give a step by step guide to the selection of controls and the movements to perform. Read the manual thoroughly, watch the video if one is provided and keep practising until you perfect the technique.

- At the end of the treatment switch off the machine.

- Remove the product, unless it is recommended to leave it on for its beneficial effects.
- Clean the electrodes.
- Dispose of waste carefully.

REMEMBER! Feedback and after care.

Clients should be encouraged to book a course of 10–12 treatments given twice a week. The timing and cost of each treatment will depend on the desired result. The client should be advised to book once or twice a month for a maintenance treatment.

SUMMARY

- Microcurrent is low intensity direct current which is modified to produce low frequency pulses of differing wave forms.

- Microcurrent is measured in microamps.

- One microamp is equal to 1/1000 of a milliamp.

summary continues overleaf

summary continued from previous page

- Microcurrents are more closely related to the body's own bio-electrical activity and help to normalize and repair damaged cells. This helps the body's own healing process.

- Current intensity is low therefore there is less stimulation of the sensory nerves, this makes the treatment less painful and more comfortable for the client.

- Machines are usually battery operated which eliminates the danger of mains electric shock.

- Machines operated from the mains have a transformer which steps down the voltage and isolates the output current, eliminating the danger of shock.

- The direct current is interrupted to produce different shaped pulses of variable duration and frequency.

- The pulse shape may be sine wave, square, rectangular, trapezoidal, triangular, saw tooth/ramp.

- Sine wave is an alternating wave form and is used for its stimulating effect on metabolism, the circulation of blood and lymph.

- Interrupted/pulsed current is used for muscle fibre stimulation, for its polar effects under the electrodes and for the metabolic and circulatory effects listed.

- Stimulation of a muscle with pulsed current will produce a muscle contraction.

- Microcurrent does not produce muscle contraction through stimulation of its motor nerve as the intensity is too low. The contraction is produced through direct stimulation of the muscle fibre, providing the intensity and duration is adequate.

- The current may be applied anywhere along the length of the fibre.

- Pulsed current will also produce polar effects under the electrodes if the pulses are flowing in one direction. Chemical reactions will occur at the cathode and anode and these effects are used in some treatments. When these effects are not required the current may be reversed between impulses, producing depolarized current.

- If the current is depolarized the chemicals formed at the electrodes during the forward wave are neutralized by the reverse wave.

- Machine controls will vary with each system. Look at the controls on the machine and make sure that you understand what each one does and how to operate it correctly. Follow the instructions in the training manual.

- Types of electrodes: adhesive electrodes, roller electrodes, probes, gloves.

- See text for effects, uses, contraindications, precautions, treatment technique.

- Recommended course of treatment: two treatments per week for 5 or 6 weeks.

- Total 10–12 treatments.

- Maintenance: one to two treatments per month.

QUESTIONS

1 Define microcurrent used in beauty therapy.

2 Explain why microcurrent is effective in improving the condition of the tissues.

3 Explain why microcurrent is more comfortable for the client than higher intensity currents.

4 Give the units of measurement of microcurrent.

5 State two ways in which the danger of mains electric shock is eliminated in microcurrent machines.

6 Give four examples of wave forms produced by microcurrent machines. Illustrate your answer with diagrams.

7 Complete the following:
Alternating current will not produce muscle contraction and is mainly used for its stimulating effects on ....

8 Explain how a muscle contraction is produced by:
(a) A faradic or higher intensity direct current.
(b) State the reason why microcurrent will not produce a contraction in the same way.

9 Explain the following terms:
(a) Polarized current.
(b) Depolarized current.

10 Complete the following:
An interrupted direct microcurrent of adequate duration and intensity will stimulate .... directly resulting in contraction of the muscle. The current is also used for its .... effects.

Chemical reactions will take place under the .... (−) and under the .... (+)

It is also used to repel .... into the skin.

11 State the functions of the following controls:
(a) Intensity control.
(b) Wave form control.
(c) Polarity control.

12 Give two factors which govern the intensity of the current given during treatment.

13 Explain briefly three ways of applying the current.

14 List six general effects of microcurrent application.

questions continues overleaf

questions continued from previous page

15 List four effects produced under the cathode and four effects produced under the anode.

16 Give six uses of microcurrent treatment.

17 Give the reasons why cotton buds with plastic holders should not be used in the probes.

Oral questions

Microcurrent treatments

1 What type of current is microcurrent?

2 Why is microcurrent treatment more comfortable for the client?

3 When would you select microcurrent treatments?

4 How does the treatment bring about its effects?

5 What factors determine the selection of wave forms?

6 How often would you recommend treatment?

10 Infra-red and Ultraviolet Treatments

OBJECTIVES

After you have studied this chapter you will be able to:

1 Explain the terms wavelength and frequency.

2 State the range wavelengths of ultraviolet and infra-red rays.

3 Explain the principles of:
   (a) refraction
   (b) reflection
   (c) absorption.

4 Explain the following laws related to radiation:
   (a) Law of Grotthus.
   (b) The cosine law.
   (c) The law of inverse squares.

5 Differentiate between the luminous and non-luminous lamps.

6 Explain the effects of infra-red rays on body tissues.

7 List the contraindications to infra-red treatments.

8 Treat the client with infra-red treatments, paying due consideration to maximum efficiency, comfort, safety and hygiene.

9 Differentiate between the three bands of ultraviolet light (UVL).

10 Explain the limit of penetration of each band.

11 Distinguish between the emission from high pressure mercury vapour lamps, overhead solariums and sunbeds.

12 Explain the effects of exposure to artificial sunlight.

13 List the contraindications in the use of sunbeds.

14 Explain the factors which determine the intensity of the reaction.

15 Treat the client with ultraviolet treatments, paying due consideration to maximum efficiency, comfort, safety and hygiene.

16 Explain the use and procedure for performing a patch test.

17 Explain the relationship between timing and distance when changing the distance of mercury vapour lamps.

Infra-red (IR) rays for heating body tissues and ultraviolet rays for promoting tanning of the skin are the radiation treatments used in beauty therapy. Both infra-red rays and ultraviolet rays are part of the electromagnetic spectrum.

Underpinning Knowledge

The electromagnetic spectrum

The electromagnetic spectrum is made up of bands of radiation with differing wavelengths and frequencies, each of which will have different physiological effects on body tissues. It is thought that all electromagnetic rays are similar in form, being particles in motion. They are transverse waves which travel through space without the need of a conductor.

The speed, or velocity, at which they travel is the same for all the bands, being 300,000 km/sec (the speed of sound).

Wavelengths of each band emitted from the spectrum

The wave band ranges are shown below, but there is some overlap.

Cosmic	up to 0.002 nm
Gamma	0.002 nm to 0.14 nm
X-rays	0.14 nm to 13.4 nm
Ultraviolet	10 nm to 400 nmm
Visible	400 nm to 770 nm
Infra-red	770 nm to 400,000 nm
Radio	100,000 nm upwards

Wavelength

The bands of the electromagnetic spectrum have different wavelengths. The wavelength is the distance between a point on one wave and the same point on the next wave.

The shortest wavelength rays are Cosmic rays and the longest are radio waves.

The distance from A to B is the wavelength. This wavelength varies from the very short wavelength of cosmic rays, measured in nanometres, to the very long wavelength of radio waves measured in metres or kilometres. (One nanometre is a very small measurement, being one millionth of a millimetre. It is written as nm.) The previous table gives the wavelengths of each band emitted from the spectrum. There is overlap between some of the bands.

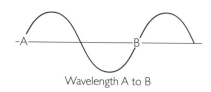

Wavelength A to B

Figure 10.1   Wavelength

number of complete waves that pass a point in one second. Many more waves of short wavelength will pass the point in one second than those of long wavelength.

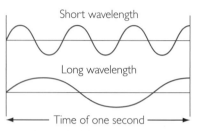

Figure 10.3 Rays of different wavelength will have different frequencies

The rays of shorter wavelength will have a higher frequency than the rays of longer wavelength. In other words, as the wavelength increases, the frequency decreases. (The term frequency is familiar to us when tuning the radio: programmes are transmitted on the radio at different frequencies.)

Units of frequency

Frequency is measured in hertz (Hz). The number of waves past a point in one second is the number of hertz, for example 50 waves passing a point per second = 50 Hz. For higher frequencies the units become

1 kilohertz (kHz) = 1000 Hz
1 megahertz (mHz) = 1000 kHz

Properties and laws of radiation

In order to give the most effective and safe treatment, the beauty therapist should be

Figure 10.2 An upright sunbed

Frequency

The bands of the spectrum also have different frequencies. Frequency is the aware of certain laws and principles which govern the behaviour of rays/waves. Both infra-red, visible light and ultraviolet rays will travel in straight lines until they meet a new medium, where they may be refracted, reflected or absorbed.

Refraction

This is the bending of rays when they meet a new medium; a common example is looking at a stick held in water – it appears to bend. Refraction occurs when rays pass from one medium to another, for example from air through glass or water. The rays striking the part are known as incident rays, or the ray of incidence. If the incident rays strike the part at right angles, they will pass straight through. If the rays strike the part at an angle, they will bend towards or away from the *normal*, depending on the medium. (The *normal* is an imaginary line which lies perpendicular to the surface.)

- If the rays pass into a more dense medium, they will bend towards the normal.
- If they pass into a less dense medium, they will bend away from the normal.

Reflection

This is the reflection of rays when they meet a surface. Shiny or white surfaces reflect more rays than dark surfaces, which absorb rays: a greater proportion of light rays will be reflected by snow than by soil. A mirror is designed to reflect rays.

The law of reflection states that the angle of incidence is equal to the angle of reflection. To measure these angles, an imaginary line is drawn perpendicular to the surface struck by the rays: this is the *normal*.

- The angle of incidence lies between the ray of incidence and the normal.

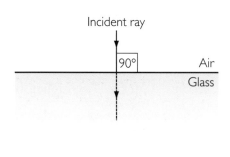

Incident ray striking the part at 90° will pass straight through

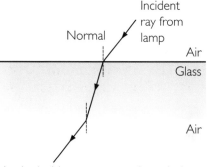

As the incident ray passes through the glass it bends towards the normal because glass is more dense. As it passes into the air again it bends away from the normal

Figure 10.4   Refraction

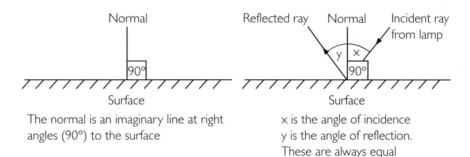

The normal is an imaginary line at right angles (90°) to the surface

x is the angle of incidence
y is the angle of reflection.
These are always equal

Figure 10.5   Reflection

- The angle of reflection lies between the ray of reflection and the normal. In Figure 10.5, X is the angle of incidence. Y is the angle of reflection. These are always equal.

The angle of incidence is one of the factors governing the proportion of rays absorbed by the medium which the rays strike. This is an important consideration when giving UV and IR treatments, as the effectiveness of the treatments will depend on the number of rays absorbed.

Absorption

The law of Grotthus states that: 'rays must be absorbed to produce an effect'.

The amount of absorption and consequently the effect depends on the following:

1 The wavelength and frequency of the rays:
  (a) Infra-red is absorbed at a level of 3 mm approximately.
  (b) Ultraviolet is absorbed at a level of 1 mm approximately.
  (This is dealt with in greater depth on page 236.)

2 The type of medium:
  (a) Certain substances absorb rays while others allow the rays to pass through (e.g. window glass absorbs most ultraviolet rays but allows visible rays to pass through).
  (b) Sunglasses are especially designed to absorb ultraviolet rays but allow visible rays to pass through. In the same way, body tissues absorb certain wavelengths at certain levels, but allow others to pass through.

3 The angle at which the rays strike the part also affects absorption. The cosine law governs the way intensity, hence absorption, is affected by the angle of incidence.

The cosine law

The cosine law states that the intensity of radiation at a surface varies with the cosine of the angle of incidence (i.e. the angle between the incident ray and the normal).

Incident ray striking the surface at 90°. There is no reflection, therefore there is maximum absorption

Figure 10.6   Cosine law

If the incident rays strike the part at 90°, there will be no angle between the incident ray and the normal (it is 0°); here there is maximum intensity and absorption. As the incident ray moves down towards the surface, the angle increases and the intensity decreases.

In Figure 10.7, X and Y are the angles of incidence. As the angle becomes greater, X to Y, the intensity at the surface decreases. The amount of decrease can be calculated by measuring the angle between the incident ray and the normal and looking up its cosine in the cosine tables.

> The cosine of 0° is 1
> The cosine of 60° is 0.5

Therefore, if the angle of incidence moves from 0° to 60°, the intensity is halved. It will diminish further as the angle increases. In order to ensure the most effective treatment, the rays must strike the part at 90°; this will ensure maximum intensity, absorption and effect, for example the sun's rays are more likely to burn at mid-day when the sun is at right angles than in the late afternoon, when it is low in the sky (if the exposure time is the same).

Intensity of radiation

The intensity of radiation will depend on three factors:

1 The intensity of the lamp.
2 The distance between the lamp and the skin.
3 The angle at which the rays strike the part.

The intensity of the lamp

Lamps vary in output and therefore, intensity; some have control dials for increasing and decreasing intensity. The intensity from infra-red lamps does not pose any problems, as the client is able to feel if the intensity is too high and the distance can be increased or the lamp turned down. However, ultraviolet rays do not give out heat and cannot be felt, therefore the distance and time of exposure must be carefully calculated to produce the

The greater the angle at y the less the intensity

Figure 10.7   Incident ray striking at different angles

required effect. This is calculated using the patch test.

The patch test procedure is only relevant when using mercury vapour lamps for treating conditions such as acne. It is not necessary to carry out this test when giving sunbed treatments.

Sunbeds are designed to emit certain intensities at their set distance and so produce the required effect in a certain time. Manufacturers' instructions should be adhered to and consideration given to sensitivity of the client (e.g. skin type and previous exposure). This is discussed fully on page 239.

The distance between the lamp and the skin

The law of inverse squares governs intensity in relation to distance.

The law of inverse squares

This law states that the intensity from a point source (i.e. the lamp) varies inversely with the square of the distance from the point source. In other words, the intensity varies inversely with the square of the distance from the source.

- If the distance increases, the intensity decreases by the square of the distance.

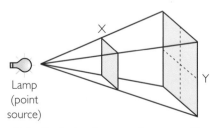

Figure 10.8 Radiation from a point source illustrating the law of inverse squares

- If the distance decreases, the intensity increases by the square of the distance.

X is one metre from the source.
Y is two metres from the source.

If the client is placed at distance X, she will receive the calculated dose. If the distance is increased to Y (i.e. doubled), then the intensity is a quarter of that at X.

REMEMBER! If you double the distance the intensity is quartered. If you reduce the distance by half, the intensity will increase four times (quadruple).

To produce the same effect on the skin when changing distances of UV lamps the following apply:

- If you halve the distance, you quarter the time.

- If you double the distance, you quadruple the time.

The angle at which the rays strike the part

The cosine law governs intensity in relation to the angle of incidence. This is fully discussed on page 226.

When giving radiation treatments, that is infra-red or ultraviolet, the lamp should be positioned so that the rays strike the part at 90°. This will ensure maximum intensity, absorption and effect.

Never position lamps directly over the client; the client should be positioned and the lamp angled so that the rays can strike at 90°.

Infra-red Rays

Infra-red rays are electromagnetic waves with wavelengths between 700 nm and 400,000 nm. They are given off by the sun and by any hot object, for example electric fires, gas and coal fires, hot packs and various types of lamps.

Figure 10.9 An infra-red lamp

The lamps that produce infra-red rays can be divided into two main types:

1 The non-luminous type (called infra-red lamps).

2 The luminous type (called radiant heat lamps).

Both these types of lamp emit infra-red rays. The difference lies in their wavelength. The non-luminous type emit rays of longer wavelength, around 4000 nm, while the luminous type emit rays of shorter wave, around 1000 nm and include waves from the visible spectrum and UVL.

The differing wavelengths produce slightly different effects when absorbed by body tissues.

> Infra-red lamps and radiant heat lamps give off (emit) infra-red rays. The difference is the wavelength of the rays which produce different effects.

The non-luminous lamps (infra-red lamps)

Many types of non-luminous lamps are produced, but they all have a non-glowing source that emits infra-red rays. A common type uses a coil of wire embedded in fireclay, which is placed in the centre of a reflector. When the lamp is switched on, the wire gets hot and heats the fireclay; the rays are then emitted from the hot fireclay, they pass through the air and are absorbed by a body placed in their path. The rays from non-luminous lamps are of longer wavelength, are invisible, are less irritating and less penetrating than the short rays from luminous lamps. They may feel hotter at equal distances and power due to increased absorption in the top layers of the skin. These wavelengths are further from visible light and are consequently called **far IR**.

The luminous lamps (radiant heat lamps)

These lamps give off infra-red rays from glowing or incandescent sources, such as

Comparisons of infra-red and radiant heat lamps

Non-luminous (infra-red)	Luminous (radiant heat)
Rays emitted from a heated wire embedded in clay	Rays emitted from glowing wires and bulbs
Long wavelength around 4000 nm	Shorter wavelength around 1000 nm
Includes no visible rays	Includes some visible rays and a small amount of UVL
Penetrates approximately 1 mm of skin to the epidermis	Penetrates approximately 3 mm of tissue to the dermis
Less irritating	More irritating
May feel hotter at equal power and distance	Will feel less hot at equal power and distance
Takes 10–15 minutes to heat up	Heats up quickly, approximately 2 minutes

hot wires or powerful bulbs. These are also placed in the centre of a reflector. When the lamp is switched on, the wire glows, giving off infra-red and visible rays and small amounts of ultraviolet rays. Some bulbs have filters to cut out some visible rays and ultraviolet rays; these bulbs are usually red in colour.

The rays produced by these lamps have a shorter wavelength, include some visible rays, are more penetrating (down to the subcutaneous layer) and are more irritating than the rays from non-luminous lamps. These wavelengths are nearer visible light and are consequently called **near IR**.

Combined infra-red and ultraviolet lamps

Manufacturers produce a wide variety of lamps, tunnels and solariums (combined UV), and you should familiarize yourself with all the lamps you find in the salon.

Some lamps have two bulbs/tubes, one producing UVL rays and the other producing infra-red rays. These lamps can be dangerous in inexperienced or incompetent hands Therapists who do not distinguish between the two may give long duration UVL by pressing the wrong switch.

- UVL glows giving a blue/white colour.
- IR gives invisible rays or glows red/orange.

Safety checks

- Examine all lamps carefully and read manufacturer's instructions.
- Check stability.
- Check joints and screws for angling the lamp; are they tight and secure?
- How can the angle of the lamp be changed?
- Is there an on/off switch on the lamp, or must it be switched on/off at the wall socket?

- Is there an intensity control, or must intensity be controlled by increasing or decreasing the distance?

- Is it in good order? Check the plugs, reflector, grid, etc.

- Is it dual purpose (i.e. infra-red and ultraviolet light)? If so make sure which switch operates infra-red and which ultraviolet.

- Is the cable sound, free from breaks in insulation and held firmly at both ends?

Infra-red Treatment to the Face

Infra-red irradiation of the face is used as a preheating treatment to prepare the skin for further treatments and aid the absorption of creams, oils and masks. Very mild heat should be given and particular attention must be paid to totally covering the eyes.

Uses

1 To soften and prepare the skin for further treatments.

2 To aid the absorption and enhance the effects of creams, oils and masks.

3 To promote healing of blemished pustular skin.

4 To open pores and aid the release of blockages.

Effects

1 Heat raises the temperature of the area and increases the metabolic rate.

2 Increase in circulation due to vasodilation.

3 Improvement of skin colour due to hyperaemia and erythema.

4 Relaxation of facial muscles.

5 Stimulation of sweat glands to produce more sweat.

6 Stimulation of sebaceous gland, releasing sebum and blockages.

Contraindications

1 Skin disorders and diseases.

2 Heavy colds or fever.

3 Migraine or headache.

4 Bruises.

5 Cuts, abrasions and chapped skin.

6 Highly sensitive skin.

7 Vascular, florid or couperosed skin as in rosacea.

8 Scars or areas of defective sensation.

9 Very dry skin, unless cream, oil, or hydrating mask is being used.

For Dangers, Precautions, Treatment technique see following text: Infra-red Treatment of the Body.

Infra-red Treatment of the Body

Infra-red is used by the beauty therapist to heat body tissues. It may be used to treat localized areas or the body in general.

Uses

1 As a general heating treatment to promote relaxation.

2 As a localized treatment for relief of pain and muscle tension.

3 As a preheating treatment, either generally or locally, to increase the circulation and thus make following treatments more effective.

Effects of infra-red irradiation

Heating of body tissues

When infra-red rays are absorbed by the tissues, heat is produced in the area. The rays from luminous generators penetrate more deeply than those from non-luminous lamps, therefore superficial and deeper tissues are heated directly. With non-luminous lamps the top 1 mm of skin is heated directly, but the deeper tissues are heated by conduction.

Increased metabolic rate

Van't Hoff's law states that a chemical reaction capable of being accelerated will be accelerated by heat.

Metabolism involves chemical reactions which will be accelerated by heat. The increase in metabolic rate will be greatest where the heating is greatest, that is in the superficial tissues; therefore more oxygen and nutrients are required and more waste products and metabolites are produced.

Vasodilation with increase in circulation

Heat has a direct effect on the blood vessels producing vasodilation and an increase in blood flow in an attempt to cool the area. Vasodilation is also produced by stimulation of sensory nerve endings which cause reflex dilation of arterioles.

Vasodilation is also produced as a result of the increase in metabolic rate and increase in waste products. The metabolites act on the walls of capillaries and arterioles causing dilation.

The heat-regulating centre of the brain will be stimulated as body heat rises. This will result in general dilation of superficial vessels to ensure that the body is not overheated. Hyperaemia is the term used to describe an increase in the flow of blood to the area due to vasodilation. Erythema means reddening of the skin due to hyperaemia and vasodilation.

Fall in blood pressure

If the superficial blood vessels dilate, the peripheral resistance is reduced and this will result in a fall in blood pressure. (When blood flows through vessels with small lumen, it exerts a certain pressure on the walls. If the lumen is increased by the vessels dilating, the pressure on the walls will be reduced.)

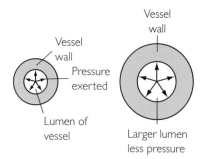

Figure 10.10   Pressure on vessel walls

A fall in blood pressure is due to the blood vessels dilating.

Increase in heart rate

The increased metabolism and circulation means that the heart must beat faster to meet the demand; therefore the heart rate increases.

General rise in body temperature

When one area of the body is heated for a prolonged time, there is a general rise in body temperature by conduction and convection. The heat will spread through surrounding tissues and will be carried by the blood circulating through the area.

Increased activity of sweat glands

As the body temperature rises, the heat regulating centres in the brain are affected. The sweat glands are then stimulated to produce more sweat in order to lose body heat. This increases the elimination of waste products.

Stimulation of sebaceous glands causes them to release more sebum.

Effects on muscle tissue

Muscle tissue is affected in two ways:

1 The rise in temperature produces muscle relaxation and relieves tension and pain.

2 When muscles are warm, they contract more efficiently than when they are cold. The increase in circulation provides the nutrients and oxygen necessary for muscle action and the removal of waste is speeded up.

Effects on sensory nerves

Heat has a soothing effect on sensory nerve endings. However, intense heat has an irritating effect.

Pigmentation

Repeated and intense exposure to infrared produces a purple or brown mottled appearance on the area. This may be due to destruction of blood cells and release of haemoglobin.

Contraindications

1 Areas of defective skin sensation and hypersensitive skin.

2 Heart conditions and blood pressure disorders (high or low).

3 Thrombosis or phlebitis or any areas of deficient circulation.

4 Heavy cold and fever.

5 Migraine and headache.

6 Skin disorders and diseases.

7 Diabetes, as skin sensitivity may be impaired.

8 Recent scar tissue (defective sensitivity).

9 Extensive bruising.

10 Recent exposure to UVL (sunburn).

11 Body infra-red would not be given in the last four months of pregnancy or first two days of a heavy period.

12 Any area where liniments or ointments have been applied.

13 Recent soft tissue injury.

Dangers

1 Burns may be caused
   (a) If the heat is too intense.
   (b) If the client is too near the lamp and fails to report overheating.
   (c) If the skin sensation is defective and the client may not be aware of overheating.
   (d) If the client touches the lamp.
   (e) If the lamp should fall and touch the client, or the bedding; over-heating of pillows and blankets can cause fire and burns.

2 Electric shock from faulty apparatus or water on the treatment area producing a short circuit.

3 Headache: irradiating the back of the neck and head or overheating by prolonged exposure may cause headache.

4 Faintness: overheating or extensive irradiation may cause a fall in blood pressure, which may cause faintness.

5 Damage to the eyes: infra-red exposure of the eyes can cause cataracts; a client should close her eyes and turn away from the lamp, wear goggles or have cotton wool over her eyes.

6 Constipation: this may occur following prolonged exposure and if water loss through sweating is not replaced by water intake.

7 Chill: this may occur if the client goes out into the cold too quickly after exposure.

Precautions

1 Clean the skin with cologne to remove sebum.

2 Ensure a safe distance of the lamp from the client. The distance depends on the client's tolerance and the output of the lamp (18–36 inches, 45–90 cm).

3 Do not place the lamp directly over the client.

4 Ensure that the lamp is stable with the head positioned over a foot if the lamp has three or five feet.

5 Ensure that the lamp is in good working order and that there are no dents in the reflector.

6 Ensure that the flexes are sound and not trailing in a walking area.

7 Check for contraindications.

8 Carry out a hot and cold sensitivity test (see page 234).

9 Protect the eyes.

10 Explain the importance of calling immediately if the client feels too hot, feels faint, nauseous or uncomfortable.

11 Warn the client not to move nearer to or touch the lamp.

12 The client should rest after treatment and not get up quickly.

> The distance of the lamp from the part will depend on:
>
> - The output of the lamp.
> - The tolerance of the client.

Treatment technique

Preparation of the client

1 Place the client in a comfortable position. When treating areas of the back, use side-lying or the recovery position, well supported by pillows. If treating knees, use half-lying position.

2 Check that all jewellery has been removed.

3 Clean the area with cologne to remove sebum.

4 Check for contraindications.

5 Explain the treatment to the client.

6 Carry out a sensitivity test using two test tubes: one filled with hot water, the other with cold water. Instruct the client to close her eyes. Carry out the test all over the area to be irradiated. Touch the client with either the hot test tube or the cold test tube at random over the area. Ask her if she feels hot or cold. (If the client cannot tell the difference between hot and cold, she has defective sensation and the treatment should not be carried out.)

7 Cover the areas not receiving treatment.

8 Warn the client that the warmth should be comfortable and to call if the heat becomes too intense.

9 Warn the client not to touch lamp or move closer to it.

> The rays should strike the part at 90° for maximum penetration, absorption and effect.

Procedure

1 Check the plug, leads and reflector.

2 Switch the lamp on, directed towards floor.
   (a) IR lamps take 10–15 minutes to reach maximum output.
   (b) Radiant heat (visible) lamps take around 2 minutes.

3 When maximum intensity is reached, position the lamp ensuring stability.

Rays strike the body part at 90°

Surface of lamp parallel with the body part

Rays strike the body part at 90°

Surface of lamp parallel with the body part

Figure 10.11   Positioning of the lamp

(If the lamp has three feet, place the head of the lamp over one of the feet, ensuring that the angle joints are secure.)

4 Make sure that the face of the lamp is parallel with the part so that the rays strike the part at 90° for maximum penetration, absorption and effect. Do not place the lamp directly above the client. (This also applies if infra-red rays are being used as a preheating treatment.)

5 Select an appropriate distance between 45–90 cms (18–36 inches). The selected distance depends on two factors:
(a) The intensity of the lamp.
(b) The client's tolerance.
(60 cm 24 inches is a good average.)

6 Ensure that the rays are not irradiating the client's face. (The lamp should not be irradiating the eyes or face of the client or the therapist.) If using infra-red rays for facial work, the eyes must be closed and covered with cotton wool.

7 Observe the client throughout the treatment.

8 Treatment time is 20–30 minutes, until the desired effect is obtained.

9 The treatment may be followed by massage or electrical treatments, but not UVL. (Infra-red given before

ultraviolet increases the sensitivity of the client and intensifies the reaction with risk of overdose.) Infra-red may be used after overexposure to UVL to reduce the reaction. The client should not rise suddenly after infra-red treatment (as the blood pressure is lowered and she may feel faint).

REMEMBER! Feedback and after care.

Do not place the lamp directly above the client: line up the part and the lamp at the same angle.

Points to consider when positioning the lamp

1 Ensure a safe but effective distance from the part.

2 Never place the lamp directly over the client. If it falls or the bulb breaks, it would cause burns to client.

3 Position the lamp so that the surface of the lamp is parallel with the part and the rays strike the part at 90° for maximum penetration, absorption and effect. This applies whenever the lamp is used.

4 Avoid irradiating the face and eyes when treating the body.

Ultraviolet Irradiation

Ultraviolet rays are part of the electro-magnetic spectrum: with wavelengths of between 10 nm and 400 nm, they lie between the violet end of the visible spectrum and X-rays. Ultraviolet rays are divided into three bands according to their wavelength:

- UVA with the longest wavelength – 315–400 nm
- UVB the middle band with wavelength – 280–315 nm
- UVC the shortest wavelength – below 280 nm

The wavelength determines the penetration and effects of the rays. The skin acts as a protective layer, which absorbs ultraviolet rays, preventing damage of deeper tissues.

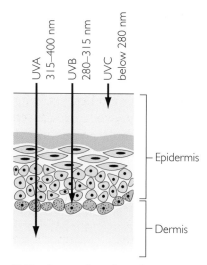

Figure 10.12   Penetration of rays into the skin

- UVA penetrates down to the capillary loops in the dermis. This causes tanning and damage to the skin's connective tissue (i.e. the elastin and collagen fibres). It may increase the risk of skin cancer.
- UVB penetrates as far as the lower levels of the epidermis – the stratum

basale. This causes tanning and also sunburn. Over exposure will cause skin cancer.

- UVC penetrates only the upper layer of the epidermis – the stratum corneum. If these rays reach the skin surface, they will damage cells and cause skin cancer. UVC rays are abiotic, they destroy bacteria.

Sources of ultraviolet radiation

1 **Natural sunlight** emits all ultraviolet rays. The intensity of UV reaching the earth's surface will vary with the time of year, the time of day, with altitude, latitude and variations in cloud cover and shade. The intensity of radiation will also increase with reflection from light surfaces, such as snow and rippling water. The destructive and harmful UVC rays are absorbed and screened out as they travel through the atmosphere; they do not reach the earth's surface. The effects of natural sunlight are therefore due to UVA and UVB. There is growing concern that as the ozone layer is becoming thinner and holes are developing; the harmful UVC rays will reach the earth.

2 **Artificial sunlight** is produced by high or low pressure tubes and lamps. In hospital departments, sun lamps are used to treat a wide variety of medical conditions. These emit UVA, UVB and some UVC rays.

In the salon, sunbeds and solariums are used for tanning the body. All the harmful UVC rays and most, if not all, of the burning UVB rays are filtered out of these beds. However, there are dangers associated with their use and operators who use them should be aware of these.

The overhead solarium

These are usually suspended at a fixed distance above the bed. They contain elements producing infra-red rays and tubes producing ultraviolet rays. They are very relaxing for the client, giving off a mild warmth and producing a tan. They emit infra-red rays, visible light, UVA, and some UVB; filters are used to control the ultraviolet emission and cut out unwanted UVB rays and all UVC rays.

There is usually an alarm clock which is set to ring half-way through the treatment to indicate that the client should turn over, and an automatic switch off at the end of the treatment. There are slight variations in the solariums available and manufacturers' instructions should be carefully studied and adhered to. Particular care must be taken with pale, sensitive-skinned clients. Worn out bulbs, tubes and filters must be replaced by the exact same models provided by the manufacturers.

Sunbeds

These come in various forms: a single bed to irradiate one side of the body or a canopy bed to irradiate both sides simultaneously. The modern beds are slightly curved to irradiate the sides of the body as well as front and back. There are stand up beds available for treatment in the standing position. The timing for treatment is greatly reduced because maintaining a standing position is very tiring. The construction of all beds is similar but the emission intensities and percentages of UVA and UVB rays differ. The beds are made up of a collection of fluorescent tubes closely packed together. The tubes are around 120 cm in length and made of vita glass, which is coated on the inside with a phosphorus lining. This lining is designed to absorb UVC rays and most if not all UVB rays. The tubes contain argon gas and some mercury with electrodes sealed at either end. When the current is switched on, the argon ionizes and electrons flow through the tube. The mercury ionizes and vaporizes and UVL is emitted. The phosphorus coating absorbs unwanted harmful rays. Some beds emit only UVA and tan slowly while others emit mainly UVA (96–98 per cent) and a small amount of UVB (2–4 per cent). These beds tan more quickly and the tan lasts longer.

The tubes are packed together side by side. There may be reflectors behind the tubes or tubes may have inbuilt reflectors so that more tubes can be incorporated into the bed giving a higher intensity of radiation.

The distance between the tubes and the surface to be irradiated is fixed and the beds are designed to produce a certain effect in a set time. The time of exposure will vary depending on the sensitivity of the client. The therapist should never assume that one sunbed is the same as another, exposure times may be different and will depend on the intensity of the radiation and skin type; manufacturer's instructions must be carefully studied and followed.

There are certain features common to all beds. They have an on/off switch and timer control; some have an emergency

Figure 10.13   A canopy sunbed

button for quick release. This should always be explained to the client and she should be able to reach the switches from the exposure position. The more modern sunbeds have a fan to control the heating.

Health and safety requirements related to sunbeds

- Instructions for use should be clearly written and displayed.

- A sunbed should always be positioned in a well-ventilated room to prevent build up of ozone which is damaging to the respiratory system and also to dissipate the heat generated by the sunbed.

- The sunbed should be isolated in its own room or behind a full-length partition so that all rays are contained and cannot irradiate other clients.

- The bed should be wiped over before and after treatment with a disinfecting detergent. Appropriate detergents supplied by the sunbed manufacturer must be used, as other detergents may damage or form a film on the acrylic surfaces, they may be toxic or inflammable, or could possibly sensitize the skin of the client.

- Sunbeds require little maintenance, but they should be regularly inspected for electrical and mechanical safety, and any faulty or exhausted tubes replaced immediately, with identical tubes supplied by the manufacturer.

Servicing and repair should be carried out by a qualified electrician in accordance with information supplied by the manufacturer.

■ The running time of the sunbed must be recorded as the tubes wear out with use and the intensity is reduced. Always check the manufacturer's instructions as the working life of tubes will vary from sunbed to sunbed. The intensity of some tubes is reduced by half after 500 hours, while others are exhausted.

■ Always replace tubes with the exact same model as the power of tubes will vary; they must be replaced by tubes of equal power and design in order to maintain radiation output. This also applies to filters.

Uses of ultraviolet irradiation

1 **Tanning (dose E1–E2)** This is the most common use in the beauty salon. It enhances appearance and gives a feeling of well-being.

2 **Tonic effect (dose E1)** UVL is thought to have a general tonic effect, improving appetite and sleep while reducing irritability and nervousness.

3 **Treatment of acne (dose E2)** Seborrhoeic skin and pustular acne benefit from UVL exposure for the following reasons:
   (a) The increase in circulation will improve the condition of the skin.
   (b) Ultraviolet has a drying effect on the skin, reducing sebum.
   (c) Desquamation following exposure will aid removal of comedones and relieve blockages.
   (d) Ultraviolet has an abiotic effect on the skin.

In hospitals, UVL is used in the treatment of wounds and ulcers, psoriasis, alopecia areata and totalis, and to produce vitamin D in the treatment and prevention of rickets.

The dangers of exposure to ultraviolet light

The effects of UV radiation on the skin will depend on the intensity of radiation and on the skin type. Dermatologists list six skin types based on skin reaction and susceptibility to sunburn.

■ **Type 1:** never tans, always burns – very sensitive.

■ **Type 2:** tans with difficulty, burns frequently – moderately sensitive.

■ **Type 3:** tans easily, burns rarely – moderately insensitive.

■ **Type 4:** always tans, never burns – moderately resistant.

■ **Type 5:** genetically brown skin (Asian or Mongoloid) – resistant.

■ **Type 6:** genetically black skin (Negroid) – very resistant.

Sunburn is an injury to the skin causing erythema, tenderness and blistering. There is no such thing as a safe level of exposure and protection against UVL is of paramount importance. The most serious effect of UVL exposure of the skin is the development of skin cancer, the most dangerous being **malignant melanoma**. Deaths from these cancers are rising every year but it is hoped that by raising public awareness of the effect of sunlight the numbers will decline.

The UK Skin Cancer Prevention Working Party has issued the following statement which will be of interest to all individuals involved with UVL treatments:

- Visible sunburn must be avoided by individuals of all ages. There is increasing evidence that excessive sun exposure and particularly sunburn when aged under 15 is a major risk factor for skin cancer in later life.

- Protection of the skin of children and adolescents is therefore particularly important.

- It is important to realize the cumulative nature of sun-induced damage particularly those who have lived abroad in sunny climates.

- Sun exposure giving rise to sunburn and skin damage can occur in the UK in Spring and Summer, therefore protection is particularly important during this time.

- Individuals who develop skin cancer do not always have a history of sunbathing. Those who have an outdoor occupation or recreational pursuits are also at risk and must protect their skin.

- There is no such thing as a safe or healthy tan. A tan is a sign that already damaged skin is trying to protect itself from further damage. The protecting power of a tan is weaker than that of a mild sunscreen with an SPF of 2–4.

- They state that four out of five cases of skin cancer are preventable.

As a result of this overwhelming evidence many local authorities, health and beauty establishments and clinics have discontinued the use of sunbeds. This would seem a very responsible course of action. However a tan is still considered desirable by many and the use of sunbeds remains popular. Awarding bodies include UVL in the electrotherapy unit, therefore it is included in this book. The decision to use a sunbed remains a matter of personal choice but everyone should be made aware of the risks.

Advice to clients

1   Individuals with fair or red hair, blue eyes and sensitive, pale skin who tan rarely and burn easily should take particular care. They should always avoid exposure to strong sunlight.

2   Prolonged exposure to sunlight, whether occupational or recreational, should be avoided.

3   Infrequent short bursts of intensive exposure must be avoided.

4   Avoid exposure between 11 a.m. and 4 p.m., when the sun is at its highest. Begin with a short exposure of 10 minutes on the first day and increase gradually each day.

5   Avoid sunbathing if taking medication (see page 246).

6   Remember that UV rays will pass through light cloud; it is, therefore, possible to burn on a cloudy day or on a sunny, windy day although it may feel cool. Keep up the protection.

7 Use every form of protection
(a) Sunscreens with a sun protection factor (SPF) of at least 15 with additional UVA protection should be used. The higher the number, the greater the protection. This sunscreen should be applied before exposure and renewed every two hours and after swimming.
(b) Cover up with a long-sleeved shirt and a hat.
(c) Find some shade under trees or some shelter.
(d) Wear polarizing sunglasses; curved ones which protect the sides as well as the front are best.

Sunbed Treatment

Guidelines for the use of sunbeds

The British Photodermatology Group have issued guidelines for those who operate and use sunbeds:

1 The use of sunbeds should not exceed two courses per year.

2 No more than ten sessions per course.

3 Each session should be timed to produce a barely perceptible erythema 8–24 hours later, and should not exceed 30 minutes per session. (This limits exposure to 10 hours per year.)

Several groups should never use sunbeds:

1 Children under 16 years.
2 People who burn easily.
3 People who do not tan or tan poorly – types 1 and 2.
4 Those taking drugs or using cosmetics which cause photosensitivity.
5 Those suffering from skin disorders aggravated by sunlight.
6 Those with a history of skin cancer.
7 Those with risk factors for cutaneous melanoma (e.g. multiple naevii, overdose in the past).

Effects of Exposure to Ultraviolet Light

As explained earlier all exposure to UVL is damaging to the body and in particular to the skin. There is no such thing as a safe and healthy tan. A tan is a sign that there is already damage to the skin.

Erythema

Erythema reaction following ultraviolet irradiation differs from the erythema reaction following infra-red irradiation in that it does not appear immediately. It takes 6–12 hours for the redness to appear, and occurs due to the irritation of cells of the epidermis.

Erythema reaction following infra-red exposure occurs because the heat produces vasodilation. More blood flows to the area and the redness appears almost immediately.

The ultraviolet rays that reach the lower levels of the epidermis (i.e. UVA and UVB) damage and destroy some of the cells. This results in the chemical histamine being released in response to the injury. The histamine causes the blood vessels to dilate, bringing an increase in blood flow and thus producing an erythema.

Further irritation will cause greater dilation and an exudation of fluid from the vessels into the tissue spaces forming blisters. Sensory nerves will be stimulated giving soreness and pain.

The greater the ultraviolet dose, the greater the irritation, therefore the more histamine will be released and the greater will be the erythema reaction. It takes some time for these processes to occur, hence the 6–12 hours before reaction appears.

There are four degrees of erythema:

- **First degree (E1):** slight reddening, no irritation, no pigmentation, fades in 24 hours, no desquamation.

- **Second degree (E2):** deeper reddening, slight irritation, slight pigmentation, fades 2–3 days, powdery desquamation.

- **Third degree (E3):** skin is very red, hot, sore and oedematous, itchy, marked pigmentation, fades 7–10 days, sheets of skin lift off.

- **Fourth degree (E4):** similar to E3 but blisters form, may be necessary to receive hospital treatment.

Erythema reaction following ultraviolet exposure occurs because cells are damaged and histamine is released. The histamine causes the blood vessels to dilate (vasodilation), more blood flows and the redness appears. It takes longer for the erythema to appear (6–12 hours).

Tanning

Tanning develops within two days of radiation. It is produced by the action of UVA and UVB on the melanocytes in the skin. Melanocytes are specialized cells found in the basal layer/stratum germinativum of the epidermis. These branching cells produce the pigment melanin and extend upwards to provide a protective cover over the living nucleated cells of the epidermis. As the pigmentation is built up, the penetration of the rays is reduced and destruction and damage of cells lessened. Melanin is formed by the action of UVA and UVB on the amino acid **tyrosine**. Two types of melanin are produced: **eumelanin**, which produces a dark brown or black colour; and **phaeomelanin**, which produces a yellowish to red colour. The variation of brown colour found in different skin types depends upon the percentages of eumelanin and phaeomelanin produced.

Tanning of the skin is produced in two ways:

1. **Immediate tanning or quick tanning** This is produced by the UVA rays wavelength 400–315 nm. These rays stimulate and darken the melanin granules already in the skin. It requires long exposure to UVA and

fades quickly within a few days. UVA will produce a tan in those individuals who tan easily (Type 3). Type 1 and 2 or areas without a previous tan may not tan.

2 **Delayed tanning** This requires a high dose of UVA, but is produced by a low dose of UVB. These rays stimulate the melanocytes to produce new dark melanin granules. Once started, this process will continue and will produce a longer-lasting tan. Therefore the most effective tanning is produced by sunbeds emitting UVA and a very low percentage of UVB. The tanning response to ultraviolet depends on the skin.

Sensitive skins burn easily but tan very slowly; some very sensitive skins will not tan at all. Types 1 and 2 should avoid using sunbeds or keep to very low exposure times of 10 minutes for the first dose and increasing by 5 minutes each session. If there is any sign of burning, further exposure should be avoided until the erythema has completely died down.

Type 3 and 4 skins of medium sensitivity burn less easily and tan more quickly. They can take a longer exposure time without burning around 15–20 minutes for the first exposure. Type 5 and 6 dark olive skins tan quickly and rarely burn and can take longer exposure times.

Thickening of the epidermis

The UVB radiation penetrates down to the stratum basale or stratum germinativum. The irritation caused to these cells produces overactivity and increased mitosis. These rapidly multiplying cells push upwards and form a marked thickening of the stratum corneum. This may become three times its normal thickness. This acts as a protection to reduce ultraviolet penetration. The dosage must, therefore, be increased with each exposure to produce the same effect, unless extensive peeling has occurred.

When using UVL for therapeutic purposes, it is sometimes necessary to maintain preset erythema doses and the length of exposure must be increased each time to produce the same effect. In order to maintain an:

- E1 the timing must be increased by 25 per cent.
- E2 the timing must be increased by 50 per cent.

This does not apply when using sunbeds for tanning purposes, although a slightly longer exposure each time will increase the depth of tanning but the erythema must have died down.

Skin peeling (desquamation)

The normal process of desquamation is accelerated due to an increase in mitotic activity of the stratum basale and migration of cells to the surface. The amount of peeling depends on the intensity of exposure and the erythema reaction.

- **First degree erythema**, peeling hardly noticeable.
- **Second degree erythema**, fine powdery flaking.
- **Third and fourth degree erythema**, marked peeling with large flakes or sheets.

Peeling reduces the protection gained by the thickened epidermis.

Production of vitamin D

Ultraviolet radiation of the skin causes a chemical reaction which converts 7-dehydro-cholesterol found in sebum into cholecalciferol, namely, vitamin D_3.

Vitamin D is necessary for the absorption of calcium and phosphorus, which play a part in the formation and growth of teeth and bones (lack of vitamin D causes rickets). Calcium is also an important factor in the blood clotting mechanism. This production of vitamin D is an important beneficial effect of ultraviolet light on the skin.

General tonic effect

General ultraviolet irradiation has a tonic effect on the body. Appetite and sleep are improved; irritability and nervousness may be reduced.

Abiotic effect

The rays of short wavelength UVC rays are abiotic rays as they destroy bacteria and micro-organisms. They are used in germicidal lamps or cabinets. These rays can be used to destroy and prevent the growth of bacteria in wounds. UVC rays are absorbed as they pass through air; therefore, they would not reach the skin from lamps placed some distance away. Special lamps called kromeyer lamps have to be used. These have enclosed tubes that are water cooled to prevent heating. They can be used in close contact with the wounds and are used in hospitals to promote healing. They are not found in beauty salons.

Therefore, the beneficial effects of UVL exposure are:

- Tanning to enhance appearance.
- Production of vitamin D, necessary for the absorption of calcium.
- Treatment of acne and psoriasis.
- General tonic effect.

Damaging effects of ultraviolet light exposure

The skin becomes dry, course, leathery, lax and wrinkled. As previously mentioned, when ultraviolet rays penetrate the skin they damage cells. UVB will damage cells down to the basal layer, as this is the limit of their penetration. UVA rays penetrate into the dermis and damage dermal cells and fibres (i.e. the elastin and collagen fibres). This produces loss of elasticity, laxity and wrinkling of the skin. Damage of cells will eventually produce thinning and dryness of the skin. Increased overactivity of some melanocytes will produce freckling and liver spots, while absence of melanocytes in other areas leave white, unpigmented patches. All these factors contribute to premature ageing of the skin. Prolonged exposure to all ultraviolet radiation should be avoided.

Carcinogenic effect

This is the most serious effect of UVL exposure of the skin

There are three main types of skin cancer:

1   Basal cell carcinoma.

2   Squamous cell carcinoma.

3   Malignant melanoma.

Malignant melanoma is the most dangerous and difficult to control.

There is indisputable evidence to link exposure to natural and artificial UVL (i.e. UVA and UVB) with skin degeneration and skin cancer. It was thought that only UVB rays were responsible, but it is now thought UVA rays may also have a carcinogenic effect. To date, the development of squamous cell carcinoma has been reported in mice exposed to UVA, but it has yet to be proven that UVA exposure alone induces carcinoma in humans.

Skin ageing (solar elastosis or photoageing)

The ultraviolet rays penetrating the skin affect the DNA in the nucleus of the cells. This interferes with the replication of the cells predisposing to skin cancer. Fair or pale skinned individuals who burn easily and tan rarely (types 1 and 2) are vulnerable as are those with multiple naevi or with previous history of severe sunburn. Long exposures to natural sunlight and prolonged frequent use of sunbeds should be avoided.

Damaging effect on the eyes

The tough outer coating of the eye called the cornea and the lens of the eye can be adversely affected by radiation. UVB and UVC rays are absorbed by the cornea and do not penetrate further. High intensity exposure to these shorter wavelengths may induce keratitis (inflammation of the cornea) and conjunctivitis (inflammation of the conjunctiva). Both these conditions are extremely irritating and painful.

The long UVA rays penetrate further and are absorbed by the lens; overexposure can cause opaqueness of the lens known as cataract.

Certain rays may penetrate down to the retina and may be a contributing causal factor for macular degeneration which may result in partial blindness in later life.

Polarizing goggles and sunglasses should always be worn in both natural and artificial sunlight. The damaging effects should be clearly explained to clients.

Polymorphic light eruption

Certain individuals react adversely to ultraviolet exposure and develop skin eruptions. The reaction occurs a few hours after exposure. There is reddening of the skin and the development of hard, itchy papules and scaling. The reaction will clear in 2–6 days, providing the skin is not exposed to further radiation.

Photosensitization

Certain drugs and cosmetics will produce photosensitization in individuals who expose themselves to the sun. A painful itchy rash develops which may be followed by pronounced permanent pigmentation. A list of these drugs appears on page 246.

Damage to the immune system

Ultraviolet radiation reduces the effectiveness of the immune system. Disturbances and reduction in the number of certain lymphocytes occur as a result of exposure to ultraviolet radiation (including UVA sunbeds). These changes, both cutaneous and systemic, diminish the response of the immune system to infections.

Aggravation of certain skin conditions

This occurs as a result of UV exposure e.g. eczema and systemic lupus erythematosus are exacerbated.

Damaging effects of UVL exposure:

- Sunburn
- Skin cancer
- Skin ageing
- Eye damage
- Impairment of immune function
- Polymorphic light eruption
- Photosensitisation

Sunbed treatments

Contraindications to sunbed and solarium treatments

1 Individuals who burn easily.

2 Individuals who do not tan easily in the sun; as these individuals have no protection, there is an increased risk of skin damage (types 1 and 2).

3 Those suffering from skin disorders aggravated by sunlight, such as eczema, dermatitis, vitiligo and chloasma.

4 Those who are unwell with colds, fever and high temperature.

5 Those with migraine, headache, faintness.

6 Those with cold sores (herpes simplex).

7 Wounds or recent scars.

8 Heart and blood pressure disorders.

9 Those undergoing or having been treated with deep X-ray therapy.

10 Those with multiple naevi or those with a naevus showing changes in size, pigmentation or inflammation, or anyone with a previous history of skin cancer.

11 Those taking drugs which may produce photosensitization, these include:

antibiotics	gold injections
tranquillizers	insulin
steroids	thyroid extract
diuretics	quinine
birth control pills	blood pressure tablets

There may be other sensitizing drugs; always seek a doctor's advice if clients are taking any medication.

12 Those on long-term immunosuppression drugs.

13 Ultraviolet exposure during pregnancy may result in uneven pigmentation (chloasma).

14 Certain treatments should not be carried out in conjunction with ultraviolet treatment, namely, epilation, waxing, and infra-red before ultraviolet exposure, as ultraviolet increases sensitivity. (However, infra-red given after ultraviolet exposure will reduce the reaction.)

Factors which determine the intensity of the reaction

The erythema reaction of a client will depend on many factors.

The sensitivity of the client

The reaction of different clients to ultra-violet varies considerably, as shown in the list of skin types (see page 239). The sensitivity of the skin also varies on different parts of the body. Exposed surfaces are less sensitive than those that are normally covered by clothing. The extensor aspects are generally less sensitive than the flexor aspects. When using sunbeds, the manufacturer's instructions should be carefully followed; first doses should be reduced for sensitive clients.

The output of the lamp or sunbed

Sunbeds are designed to produce a required reaction at a set distance in a certain time. Tubes should be replaced regularly and if damaged in order to maintain the same output.

The higher the output of the sunbed the greater the reaction in a set time. Always set the times according to the manufacturers' instruction.

The duration of exposure

The duration of exposure will have an effect on the reaction. The longer the time, the greater the reaction at a constant distance.

The distance between the lamp or tubes and the client

The nearer the lamp or the shorter the distance from the surface, the greater the reaction. Again this does not apply to sunbeds where distance is constant.

The angle at which the rays strike the part (angle of lamp)

The angle at which the rays strike the skin affects the dosage. According to the cosine law, maximum absorption takes place when the rays strike the skin at right angles. Sunbeds are designed with reflectors to focus the rays on the area and angles cannot be changed.

Previous exposure of the area

An exposure should not be repeated until the previous erythema has faded, as until this occurs sensitivity is increased. When the erythema has faded, there will be a thickening of the skin. It is, therefore, necessary to increase exposure in order to repeat the reaction on the same area of skin. If there has been marked peeling, the exposure should be decreased.

Infra-red irradiation applied before exposure to ultraviolet radiation increases the erythema reaction. Infra-red applied after ultraviolet reduces the effects. Simultaneous irradiation with both types of ray does not affect the reaction.

Precautions

1 On the first consultation, discuss the following with the client:
    (a) Skin type, i.e. fair, medium or dark skinned?
    (b) Reaction to sunlight, i.e. does the client goes red and never tans, goes red first then tans, or rarely goes red but tans easily?
    (c) Ask when the last exposure to sunlight was received.

The timing of the first dose will depend on these factors.

2   Check for contraindications.

3   Explain the procedure to the client; show her the switch, timer, release button and other facilities. Show the client how to get on and off the bed.

4   Explain the importance of calling for help if the client feels faint, nauseous, too hot or suffers skin irritation.

5   Explain the importance of wearing the goggles provided.

6   Explain the importance of not exceeding the treatment time.

7   Always maintain high standards of hygiene.
    (a) The client must shower, both for cleanliness and to remove lotions and perfumes.
    (b) Provide a disposable floor covering for each client.
    (c) Clean the sunbed before and after treatment with detergent recommended by manufacturer.

8   Check the reaction to the previous dose.

9   Keep a careful record of the date and timing of treatment and check the reaction on next visit.

Treatment technique

Preparation of sunbed

1   Ensure that the sunbed is in good working order.

2   Check and set the switch, timer, etc.

3   Clean the bed with a disinfecting detergent recommended by the manufacturer.

4   Place a clean disposable floor covering for each client.

5   Provide clean towels for each client.

6   Provide clean goggles for each client. Disposable goggles must be provided or the client may keep her own.

7   Ensure that the sunroom is well ventilated.

Preparation of client

1   Check for contraindications.

2   Remove all make-up.

3   Remove all jewellery.

4   Shower using non-perfumed soap to remove perfume, cologne, lotions and ointments as these may produce photosensitization.

5   Ensure that the skin is dry.

6   Remove contact lenses.

7   Wear protective goggles (curved polarizing).

8   Cover hair, particularly coloured and bleached hair.

9   Protect protruding haemorrhoids.

10 Do *not* apply any suntan oils or lotions.

11 For sunbeds, the first dose should not exceed 15 minutes – do not give a second dose if there was adverse reaction, such as fainting, nausea, intense irritation, rash or intense erythema. Do not give further treatment until all erythema has subsided.

12 Stay in easy reach of the client and show her how the sunbed works and how to operate the release button. Explain the dangers of not heeding contraindications and not wearing goggles, etc.

13 After each session, advise the client to get up slowly and apply moisturiser to her face and body.

14 Keep a careful record of: the date of treatment, timing of treatment and reaction to treatment.

Dermatologists recommend that exposure to ultraviolet rays should not exceed 10 hours per year – two courses of 10 half-hour sessions.

REMEMBER! Feedback and after care.

Local Council Regulations in Relation to Infra-red and Ultraviolet Treatments

Any salon offering infra-red or ultraviolet treatments must adhere to the local authority regulations.

Construction of equipment

The collapse of any ultraviolet tanning equipment may give rise to electric shock, fire, or direct physical injury. Equipment should therefore be of adequate mechanical strength and rigidity. Lamps should be adequately protected by embedding them within reflectors, or by covering them with a grille mesh.

Layout

- To facilitate rapid entrance or exit from a cubicle containing the equipment, any door should be fitted so that its opening cannot be impeded and must be able to be opened from the outside. Equipment must be designed for easy release by the user.

- Ensure adequate ventilation is provided to prevent a build up of ozone and to ensure that heat generated by the bed is adequately dissipated.

- If the ultraviolet tanning equipment is not in individual cubicles, then suitable screens or curtains should be provided to prevent unnecessary exposure to other persons.

Washing facilities

Showering/washing facilities should be provided for hygiene reasons.

Cleaning the equipment

Surfaces that come into contact with clients should only be cleaned with the appropriate cleaning agents. Other agents may damage or form a film on the acrylic surface; they may be toxic or inflammable or could sensitize the skin of the client.

Exposure

The operator should ensure that each client is advised of a suitable exposure regime, taking into account skin types, previous exposures and enhanced sensitivity. A good quality, reliable, automatic time switch should be carefully pre-set to terminate the exposure.

Protective eye wear

Excessive exposure of the eyes to infra-red or ultraviolet rays will result in eye damage. Provide special goggles, but ensure they are disposable or that clients keep their own pairs, to eliminate the risk of eye infections.

Maintenance

Records should be kept by the operator of all servicing and these should be available on the premises. Servicing and repair must be carried out by a qualified electrician in accordance with manufacturers' instructions. Faulty equipment must not be used. All parts must be replaced by the exact same model.

Staff training

The operator should ensure that properly trained staff are available to provide adequate advice, supervision and assistance to clients.

SUMMARY

- The electromagnetic spectrum is made up of bands of different wavelengths and frequencies. Infra-red radiation and ultraviolet radiation are part of the spectrum; they lie on either side of visible light.
- Infra-red rays are used to heat body tissues.
- Ultraviolet rays are used to tan the skin.
- All rays travel in straight lines until they meet a new medium where they may be refracted, reflected or absorbed.
- Refraction means the bending of rays towards or away from the normal as they enter a new medium.
- Reflection means that rays will reflect off certain surfaces; a greater proportion of rays are reflected from white surfaces than from dark/black surfaces.
- Absorption means that rays are absorbed by certain mediums: they do not pass through. When giving infra-red or UVL treatments, rays must be absorbed to produce and effect (law of Grotthus). The amount of absorption depends on three factors:
  1 The wavelength and frequency of rays.
  2 The type of medium.
  3 The angle at which the rays strike the part.
- The cosine law describes the way that intensity is governed by the angle of incidence. The cosine law states that the intensity at a surface varies with the cosine of the angle of incidence.

summary continues overleaf

summary continued from previous page

- The intensity at surface depends on:
  1 The intensity of the lamp.
  2 The distance between the lamp and the skin.
  3 The angle at which the rays strike the part.
- Rays should strike the part at 90° for maximum intensity, absorption and effect.
- The law of inverse squares governs intensity in relation to distance. The law of inverse squares states that the intensity from a point source varies inversely with the square of the distance from the source. If you halve the distance, you must quarter the time. If you double the distance, you quadruple the time.
- Both infra-red lamps (non-luminous) and radiant heat lamps (luminous) emit infra-red rays, the difference lies in their wavelength. See page 222 for the differences.

Dangers of infra-red treatment
1 Burns.
2 Shock.
3 Headache.
4 Faintness.
5 Eye damage.
6 Chill.

NOTE! Always carry out a skin sensitivity test before applying infra-red to the body. The client must be able to distinguish between hot and cold. Use two test tubes, one with hot water and the other with cold water. Instruct the client to close her eyes. Touch the area to be irradiated with either the hot or cold test tube and ask the client to say if it feels hot or cold. A failure to identify the hot or cold test tube means that treatment should not be carried out.

Ultraviolet
- Ultraviolet rays are used for tanning the body and for certain conditions, such as acne and psoriasis. Ultraviolet rays are divided into three bands according to their wavelength:
  1 UVA – the longest wavelength, penetrates down to the dermis. Damages elastin and collagen, causes premature ageing and can cause cancer. Quick tanning, quick fading.
  2 UVB – middle wavelength, penetrates to stratum basale. Causes sunburn and cancer. Slow tanning, longer lasting.
  3 UVC – shortest wavelength, penetrates the stratum corneum. Cell damage and cancer. Abiotic rays destroy micro-organisms.
- Emission of ultraviolet rays from natural sunlight include all three, but all the UVC and some UVB are filtered out in the atmosphere and do not reach the earth's surface.

summary continues overleaf

summary continued from previous page

- UVC are dangerous and destructive rays. They destroy bacteria and are known as abiotic or germicidal.

- UVB rays are burning rays. They are responsible for sunburn due to overexposure. Long-term or intense exposure to UVB can cause skin cancers.

- At one time it was thought that UVA rays would tan without producing harmful effects. However, they penetrate more deeply into the skin and damage the connective tissue in the dermis, damaging collagen and elastin fibres which causes ageing and wrinkling of the skin. There is also increasing evidence that intense and over exposure to UVA can cause certain skin cancers.

- Artificial UVL is produced by lamps and tubes found in solariums and sunbeds.

Solariums

- These contain elements emitting infra-red and tubes emitting UVL. All UVC and most UVB are filtered out of solariums.

Sunbeds

- These are composed of a collection of long tubes which emit mainly UVA and may also emit very small amounts of UVB.

- Exposure to artificial sunlight will produce some beneficial effects on the body. However, great care must be taken as over or prolonged exposure will have very undesirable effects. (These are fully discussed on page 244.)

- Instructions for use must be clearly written and displayed.

- Contraindications to use of sunbeds must be very carefully studied (see page 246).

- Hygiene precautions when using sunbeds:
  1 Clients should shower and dry before use.
  2 The sunbed should be cleaned with a recommended detergent before and after treatment.
  3 Provide a disposable floor covering.
  4 Provide disposable goggles.
  5 Provide clean towels for each client.
  6 Ensure that the room is well ventilated.

- Before exposure discuss with the client:
  1 Skin type: fair, medium or dark.
  2 Reaction to sunlight (i.e. type 1, 2, 3, 4, 5 or 6).
  3 When previous dose was received.
  4 Check for other contraindications; particularly ask about any medication being taken.

- Stop the treatment if the client feels faint, nauseous or suffers from skin irritation.

- Explain the dangers of overexposure or prolonged exposure.

- Guidelines for users and operators of sunbeds:
  1 Use of sunbeds should be limited to two courses a year.
  2 No more than 10 sessions per course.

summary continues overleaf

summary continued from previous page

3 Each session should be timed to produce a barely perceptible erythema 8–24 hours later. The length of time of exposure should not exceed 30 minutes per session. (Exposure per year should not exceed 10 hours.)

Effects of ultraviolet exposure
1 Erythema.
2 Tanning.
3 Thickening of epidermis.
4 Skin peeling.
5 Production of vitamin D.
6 Abiotic effect of short rays (not present in normal lamps, solariums and sunbeds).
7 General tonic effect.
8 Skin ageing and wrinkling.
9 Cancer forming.
10 Damage to eyes.
11 Polymorphic light eruptions.
12 Photosensitization.
13 Damage to immune system.
14 Aggravation of certain skin conditions (e.g. eczema).

Feedback
For IR, examine the area and ask appropriate questions to obtain feedback; this will indicate if the treatment is effective and suitable and if the client is happy. For UVL, ask the client to watch for the erythema about 6 hours after treatment. This should be first degree – slight reddening.

After care
Give advice on after care and any routine to follow before next treatment.

QUESTIONS

1 Explain what is meant by:
   (a) Wavelength of rays.
   (b) Frequency of rays.
2 Define the term 'incidence ray'.
3 Where does the 'angle of incidence' lie?

questions continues overleaf

questions continued from previous page

4   Explain why a stick looks bent when held in water.

5   Define the law of Grotthus.

6   Name three factors which affect the amount absorption by a medium.

7   State the law that governs the way intensity is affected by the angle of incidence.

8   State the law that governs intensity in relation to distance.

9   List the three factors which will affect the intensity felt by a client receiving infra-red treatment.

10   Give three differences between luminous and non-luminous infra-red lamps.

11   Some lamps are manufactured with two elements, one emitting infra-red and the other ultraviolet; explain the danger when using these lamps.

12   Why must a sensitivity test be carried out before an infra-red treatment?

13   Explain the procedure for carrying out a sensitivity test.

14   Give the two factors that govern the choice of distance when giving infra-red treatments.

15   Explain why it is desirable for rays to strike the part at 90°.

16   Give three ways in which vasodilation is produced during heat treatments.

17   Explain why blood pressure will fall when giving heat treatments.

18   Explain why the heart rate increases.

19   Explain why sweating is induced during heat treatments.

20   Explain why the following are contraindications to infra-red treatments:
     (a) Heart conditions.
     (b) Thrombosis.
     (c) Headaches.
     (d) Recent exposure to UVL.

21   Give four dangers of infra-red irradiation.

22   List six precautions to be taken when giving infra-red treatments.

23   List the three bands of rays in ultraviolet light.

24   Discuss the wavelength and compare the depth of penetration of the skin by each band.

25   List six contraindications to ultraviolet irradiation.

26   Explain the procedure when preparing a sunbed for use.

27   Give three questions that would be asked of a client to determine the length of first exposure.

28   Give three beneficial effects and three detrimental effects of exposure to UVL.

29   Explain how and why tanning of the skin is one effect of exposure to UVL.

30   Give the exposure guidelines for operators and users of sunbeds to follow.

questions continues overleaf

questions continued from previous page

Oral questions

Infra-red and radiant heat treatments to face and body

1 When would infra-red/radiant heat be used?
2 Explain the difference between infra-red lamps and radiant heat lamps.
3 Explain what happens in the tissues when the body is heated.
4 Are there any dangers associated with infra-red treatment?
5 What action would you take if you found any contra-actions?
6 What factors determine where you position the lamp?
7 What is a good average distance to start from?
8 Which law governs the intensity in relation to the angle of the rays?
9 Which law governs intensity in relation to the distance of the lamp?
10 How long would the treatment last?
11 Why must infra-red never be followed by ultraviolet treatment?
12 What advice would you give the client after treatment?

Ultraviolet treatment

1 How many bands are there in the ultraviolet part of the electromagnetic spectrum?
2 Do ultraviolet rays from the sun heat the tissues?
3 Do ultraviolet rays from sunbeds heat tissues?
4 Which rays emitted from sunbeds are used for cosmetic purposes?
5 Why is ultraviolet light (sunbeds) used in the salon?
6 Does ultraviolet treatment have any other beneficial effects?
7 Which rays are abiotic rays?
8 Why and how does the skin tan when exposed to ultraviolet rays?
9 How does exposure to ultraviolet light increase the production of vitamin D?
10 Why is vitamin D production an important beneficial effect of ultraviolet exposure?
11 Give five damaging effects of ultraviolet light which give cause for great concern.
12 List the health and safety regulations relating to sunbeds.
13 What action would you take if you established that the client was taking drugs and requested sunbed treatment?
14 How would you advise a pregnant client who requested ultraviolet treatment?
15 How would you prepare the client for sunbed treatment?
16 Why is it important to remove all lotions, perfume or perfumed soap prior to treatment?
17 How would you prepare the sunbed prior to treatment?

11 Heat Therapy Treatments

OBJECTIVES

After you have studied this chapter you will be able to:

1 Differentiate between the methods of giving general heat and local heat to the body.

2 List the effects of heat on the body.

3 Explain the contraindications to heat on the body.

4 Discuss the advantages and disadvantages of steam baths and steam rooms.

5 Explain the uses of steam baths and steam rooms.

6 Select either a steam bath or steam room and treat the client, paying due consideration to maximum efficiency, comfort, safety and hygiene.

7 Briefly explain the production of dry heat in a sauna.

8 Describe the temperature range and seating advice suitable for a client using the sauna for the first time.

9 List the dangers of sauna bath treatment.

10 Treat the client using a sauna bath, paying due consideration to maximum efficiency, comfort, safety and hygiene.

11 Briefly describe the facial steamer.

12 Describe the uses of facial steamers.

13 Explain the danger of facial steamers.

14 Treat the client, paying due consideration to maximum efficiency, comfort, safety and hygiene.

15 Indicate the uses of wax treatments to identified areas of the face and body.

16 List the contraindications to wax treatments in the following areas:
(a) Hands and feet.
(b) Body.
(c) Face.

17 Prepare a wax bath and bring to the correct temperature.

18 Treat the client with wax to hands and feet; to the body; and to the face, paying due consideration to maximum efficiency, comfort, safety and hygiene.

19 Describe the care and maintenance of wax baths.

Figure 11.1   A sauna in use

Figure 11.1 is a photograph of a sauna bath; this is one method of applying general heat to the body. Many forms of heat therapy are available to the beauty therapist, and choice is determined by availability, client preference and suitability. All forms of heat produce similar effects; the treatment is particularly beneficial when combined with other treatments as part of a routine. It is mainly used before other treatments as it increases tissue response.

Heat therapy is used for the following reasons:

1 To heat the body prior to other treatments.

2 To induce muscle relaxation.

3 For relief of pain.

Heat Application

Applying general heat

1 Sauna.

2 Steam bath, steam room (e.g. Turkish and Roman baths).

3 Jacuzzi/spa pool.

4 Infra-red covered in previous Chapter 10.

5 Wax applied to the body.

6 Various forms of showers.

7 Foam bath.

Applying local heat

1 Infra-red and radiant heat lamps.

2 Paraffin wax to specific areas.

3 Whirlpool bath.

4 Facial steamers.

Effects of heat on the body

(For a detailed explanation see page 231.)

1 A general rise in body temperature.

2 An increase in blood flow to the area due to vasodilation giving hyper-aemia and erythema.

3 An increase in the heart rate/pulse rate.

4 A lowering of blood pressure.

5 An increase in the metabolic rate, therefore there is an increased demand for oxygen and nutrients and increased output of waste products.

6 Relaxation of muscles.

7 Mild heat has a soothing effect on sensory nerve endings, but intense heat is irritating to sensory nerve endings.

8 Increased activity of sweat glands (diaphoretic effect).

Heat may be applied generally or locally and the extent of the effects will be dependent on:

1 The duration of heat application.

2 The intensity or degree of the heat.

3 The depth of absorption.

4 The size of area being heated.

Contraindications to general heat therapy

1 Areas of defective sensation and hypersensitive skins.

2 Heart conditions and blood pressure disorders.

3 Thrombosis or phlebitis.

4 Bronchitis, asthma, hay fever or heavy colds and fevers.

5 Migraine and headache.

6 Skin disorders, such as eczema and psoriasis, but these may be helped by wet heat (with medical approval).

7 Diabetes.

8 Epilepsy.

9 After a heavy meal.

10 Under the influence of alcohol or drugs.

11 Later stages of pregnancy.

12 First 1–2 days of a period, especially if it is heavy.

13 Severe exhaustion.

14 Recent overexposure to UVL (e.g. sunburn).

Steam Treatments

- Steam may be applied to the body using steam baths or steam rooms. It may be applied to the face by means of facial steamers.

- Steam treatments applied to the body promote relaxation, have a deep cleansing effect and make the tissues more receptive to following treatments.

- Steam is used on the face to soften the skin for deep cleansing and to aid the absorption of creams, oils and masks.

Figure 11.2   A rigid arm vapouriser for facial steam treatment

Facial Steam Treatment

Steam may be applied to the face using floor standing or table facial vaporizers. Some vaporizers deliver steam only, while others deliver steam and ozone. (Ozone is known to be damaging to the respiratory tract and is not medically recommended. Although only very small amounts are produced by vapour/ozone steamers and the timing of the treatment is reduced to 5 minutes, therapists should take care when giving this treatment.)

The facial steamer consists of a tank with a heating element. This is filled with distilled water, which is heated, producing steam. This steam passes into a tube, which is directed at the client's face. If it produces ozone, the steamer will contain a high pressure mercury vapour tube producing ultraviolet rays. This converts the oxygen in the air into ozone (i.e. O_2 is converted into O_3). Facial steamers produce heating with high humidity.

Uses

1 To soften superficial keratinized cells and build-up of sebum on seborrhoeic greasy skin prior to desquamation and deep cleansing.

2 To aid absorption and enhance the effect of creams, oils and masks, etc. Used to improve the condition of dry, dehydrated and normal or mature skins.

3 To promote relaxation.

4 To prepare the skin for further treatments.

5 To aid healing of blemished or pustular seborrhoeic skins.

Effects

1 The heat raises the temperature of the area.

2 The circulation is increased due to vasodilation, giving hyperaemia and erythema.

3 The heat induces muscle relaxation.

4 Mild heat is soothing to sensory nerve endings.

5 The heat increases the metabolic rate.

6 Sweat glands are stimulated producing more sweat (diaphoretic effect).

7 Sebaceous glands are stimulated, opening pores and aiding the release of blockages.

8 If ozone is used, it has a bactericidal effect.

Contraindications

1 Highly vascular florid or couperosed skin.

2 Highly sensitive skin (low heat tolerance) or telangiectasis.

3 Very dry or weathered skin.

4 Rosacea.

5 Abrasions or chapped skin.

Dangers

1 Burns if the steamer falls over on to the client.

2 Shock if the apparatus is faulty.

3 Damage to the respiratory tract if too much ozone is inhaled.

Ensure that the tank contains distilled water.

Precautions

1 Check that there is distilled water in the tank.

2 Switch on for 5–10 minutes before treatment until the vapour is produced.

3 Switch on the ozone after the production of vapour.

4 Cover the client's eyes with damp cotton wool pads.

5 Make sure that the steamer is positioned safely so that it cannot be overturned, causing burns.

6 Make sure that the steamer is working correctly and not spitting out hot water.

If using vapour ozone remember that ozone can damage the respiratory system. Ensure that the steamer is 46 cm/18 inches from the face and timing reduced to 5 minutes.

Treatment technique

Preparation of the client

1 Place the client in a comfortable, well-supported position.
2 Remove all jewellery and metals.
3 Check for contraindications.
4 Cover all areas except the face with towels.
5 Cleanse the skin.
6 Explain the procedure to the client.
7 Apply cotton wool pads to the client's eyes.

Procedure

1 Place the machine in a stable position and check the plugs and leads.
2 Fill the tank with distilled water. This is important because minerals etc. in the water can impair the function of the equipment.

3 Switch on and allow the steam to build up, then switch on the ozone if required.
4 Position 38–46 cm/15–18 inches from the client's face, depending on skin type and tolerance.
5 Time 5–20 minutes depending on the required effect. (If vapour ozone is used, timing should be reduced to 5 minutes and the distance increased to 46 cm/18 inches.)
6 Switch off and remove the machine to a safe place.
7 Dry the skin and remove the eye pads.
8 Extract any comedones, milia, etc.
9 Follow with other treatments.

Facial steam treatment time	Distance from face
Greasy seborrhoeic skin	15–20 mins at 38 cm/15 inches
Normal skin	10–15 mins at 38 cm/15 inches
Dry mature skin	3–7 mins at 38–46 cm/15–18 inches

REMEMBER! Feedback and after care.

Body Steam Treatments

The steam bath

This bath is designed for individual treatments. It is a cabinet made of moulded fibreglass in which the client sits. It contains a trough with a heating element; water poured into the trough is heated making steam. The trough is placed underneath an adjustable seat which allows the client to sit comfortably with her head outside the bath. There are usually three controls: a main switch, a timer and temperature gauge. The water is heated, forming steam which condenses within the bath and the air is saturated with very high humidity of around 95 per cent.

The steam room

This is a room which is supplied with steam from a boiler. Several people may use the steam room together. Some complexes based on Turkish baths have several rooms with increasing temperatures. Clients start with the lowest temperature and progress through to the highest. The steam bath has several advantages over the steam room. However, group treatments in steam rooms are more sociable occasions.

Advantages of the steam bath over the steam room

1 The client does not feel claustrophobic because her head is out of the bath.

2 The clients breathe normal air and not steam.

3 The hair remains neat and tidy and does not get wet.

4 The bath offers privacy for the client.

5 The temperature can be adjusted to suit the individual.

6 The initial cost and the running cost is low compared with a steam room.

7 It takes up little space and can be accommodated in most salons.

8 It is easier to clean thus ensuring high hygiene standards and reducing the risk of cross infection.

Uses

1 To prepare client for further treatment.

2 To induce relaxation.

3 For deep cleansing.

Effects of steam heat

1 A general rise in body temperature.

2 An increase in circulation due to vasodilation giving hyperaemia and erythema.

3 The heart/pulse rate increases.

4 Superficial capillaries and vessels dilate; therefore, there is a fall in blood pressure.

5 An increase in cell metabolism.

6 Stimulation of sweat glands with increased sweating and elimination of waste. There may be a temporary loss of body fluid due to sweating, but this is soon adjusted by drinking water.

7 The increased circulation and rise in temperature promote muscle relaxation.

8 The mild heat soothes sensory nerve endings.

9 The superficial layer of the skin is softened and is removed more easily, improving tone and texture.

Contraindications

1   Heart and circulatory conditions.

2   High or low blood pressure.

3   Thrombosis and phlebitis.

4   Headaches, migraines, dizziness, faintness.

5   Skin diseases.

6   Athlete's foot and verrucas.

7   Diabetes, epilepsy.

8   Any chest conditions (e.g. asthma, bronchitis).

9   First days of menstruation.

10 Pregnancy.

11 After a heavy meal or drinking alcohol.

12 Clients on low calorie slimming diets.

Dangers

1   Overheating causing fainting or dizziness.

2   Burns from touching the hot metal trough.

3   Cross infection by micro-organisms.

Precautions

1   Ensure good standards of hygiene as moist heat is an ideal breeding ground for micro-organisms. Wipe over the whole bath with sterilizing detergent before and after treatment. Cover the seat and floor with towels that are boiled after use or disposed of.

2   Check the power supply and terminals are correctly switched on.

3   Check that the trough is full of distilled water.

4   Protect the client from direct contact with metal and steam using a towel.

5   Offer the client a drink of water after treatment to rehydrate.

6   Remove jewellery, glasses, contact lenses, etc.

7   Check for contraindications, particularly foot infections.

8   Ensure that the client takes a shower before and after treatment.

9   Explain the treatment to the client and demonstrate how to open the door and get out of the bath.

10 Wrap a towel around her neck to prevent steam escaping.

11 Stay within calling distance of the client and observe her frequently. Stop the treatment if the client feels faint, nauseous or too hot.

Treatment technique

Preparation of the bath before the client arrives

1   Wipe over with sterilizing detergent.

2   Fill the trough with water.

3   Protect the client from contact with hot metal and direct steam by covering the seat with a towel that hangs over the edge.

4   Place a towel over the aperture to prevent loss of steam.

5 Turn on the main switch and bath switch.

6 Turn the controls to maximum until the water is heating and then adjust the temperature and timer (50–55 °C); the bath will take around 15 minutes to heat from cold.

Figure 11.3   Preparation of a steam bath

Procedure

1 Supply the client with a gown and paper slippers.

2 Remove all jewellery, glasses, contact lenses, etc.

3 Check for contraindications.

4 Explain the treatment to the client and show her how to enter and leave the steam bath/room.

5 Help the client into the shower.

6 After the shower, help the client into the bath; make sure that she is comfortable; close the door.

7 Place a towel around the client's neck over the aperture.

8 Keep in verbal contact throughout, reassure the client and ask her to report any discomfort.

9 Treatment time is 15–20 minutes.

10 Help the client from the bath and into the shower.

11 Advise the client to use a friction rub to aid desquamation and improve skin texture.

12 The client should now rest for 20–30 minutes or receive further treatments *but not exercise*.

REMEMBER! Feedback and after care.

Sauna Baths

These baths are pinewood log cabins heated by electric stoves. They are manufactured in various sizes, from a single person sauna up to large cabins for 10–14 people. In Scandinavian countries, they are found indoors and outdoors. The larger the sauna, the more expensive it will be to run as it will require more heat output from larger stoves.

The walls of the cabin are constructed of well-insulated panels of pinewood. Pinewood allows the interchange of air and absorbs moisture. This will reduce the humidity inside the cabin, giving a dry heat. The heat is provided by electric stoves, which heat non-splintering stones placed on top of the stove. Slatted wooden benches are arranged inside the sauna for sitting or lying down. There is an air inlet near the floor and an outlet near the ceiling. As the air in the sauna is heated, it rises by convection; therefore, the sauna is hotter on the upper benches than on the lower benches. The air moisture is absorbed by the walls, making humidity very low at around 10 per cent. This humidity can easily be increased by pouring water on the stones which boils and creates steam. Because the humidity in the sauna is low, sweat from the body evaporates quickly, cooling the body, therefore high temperatures can be tolerated in the sauna. The temperature in the sauna may range from 50°C to around 120°C. A temperature range between 60–80°C is recommended for clients unfamiliar with sauna baths. This can be increased as the client's tolerance increases. The thermometer should always be checked for the temperature and the hygrometer should be checked for humidity before the commencement of treatment; these are found on a wall inside the cabin. The temperature should range from 60–80°C and the humidity should range from 50–70 per cent.

The choice between steam and sauna as a preheating treatment depends very much on the client's preference; there are certain differences to consider (see page 267).

Uses

1   Mainly used as a preheating treatment.

2   To induce relaxation.

3   For deep cleansing.

Effects

1   A general rise in body temperature.

2   An increase in circulation.

3   The heart rate increases.

4   Superficial capillaries dilate, therefore there is a fall in blood pressure.

5   Erythema is produced.

6   An increase in cell metabolism.

7   Increased sweating with elimination of waste (diaphoretic effect).

8   Produces relaxation.

9   Sedatory effect on nerve endings.

10   If sweating is excessive, it can produce dehydration.

11   The dry heat is irritating and drying to mucous membranes.

Contraindications

1   Heart and circulatory conditions.

2   High and low blood pressure.

3   Thrombosis, phlebitis.

4   Headaches, dizziness, migraines, faintness.

5   Skin diseases.

6   Athlete's foot, verrucas.

7   Diabetes, epilepsy.

8   Chest conditions (e.g. asthma, bronchitis).

9   First days of menstruation.

10   Pregnancy.

11   After heavy meals or alcohol intake.

12   Clients on low calorie diets.

Dangers

1   Fainting or dizziness if blood pressure falls too low.

2   Dehydration with prolonged and frequent treatments.

3   Dryness and irritation of mucous membranes (e.g. the throat and nose).

The therapist should supervise the sauna and stop the treatment if the client feels faint, giddy or nauseous.

> Clients must be instructed to come out of the sauna if they are feeling unwell, if they feel faint, nauseous, dizzy or overheated. The therapist must always remain close at hand to help when necessary.

Precautions

1   Check the temperature (60–80 °C) and humidity (50–70 per cent) before use.

2   Check that the guard around the heating element is secure and in position.

3   The client must shower to remove all make-up, perfumes, etc.

4   Ensure that the client removes contact lenses, glasses and jewellery.

5   Examine the client for contraindications, particularly the feet for athlete's foot and verrucas.

6   Use disposable slippers and paper on the floor.

7   Observe the client throughout treatment and check the time.

8   Boil towels or robes after each treatment.

9   Scrub the benches and floor thoroughly with special disinfectant for saunas after use.

10   Ensure that there is water available for the client; explain the importance of drinking water for rehydration.

Treatment technique

1   Prepare the sauna before the client arrives. Protect the floor with paper towelling and bench with towels.

2   Explain the procedure to the client and stress that she must come out if she feels dizzy or faint. Check for contraindications.

3   The client should shower before treatment and remove jewellery, contact lenses and glasses.

4   The client should wear some form of hair protection.

5   The client enters the sauna with or without a towel wrap and wears disposable slippers.

6   Advise the client to sit or lie on the lower benches until she is accustomed to the heat (hot air rises; lower benches are at lower temperature).

7   Small amounts of water may be sprinkled on the stones from time to time to increase the humidity (this should not be overdone).

8 Treatment time will depend on the tolerance of the client. The first treatment could be up to 5 minutes, increasing to 14 minutes or 20 minutes as the tolerance is built up.

9 Warm or cold showers may be taken during the course of the treatment.

10 The client must always shower after a sauna.

11 Rest after treatment or continue with other treatments, for example massage or vacuum suction, but no exercise.

12 Scrub benches and floor thoroughly with special disinfectants.

REMEMBER! Feedback and after care.

Differences between steam baths and saunas

Steam	Sauna
Moist heat, humidity 95 per cent	Dry heat, humidity 50–70 per cent
Atmospheric air is inhaled, therefore more suitable for clients with mild respiratory problems	Hot, dry air is inhaled which may irritate the mucous membranes
Easily adjusted to the tolerance of individual clients	Usually communal, therefore difficult to adjust to the needs of individual clients
Not claustrophobic as the head is free	May be claustrophobic
Not as damaging to hair as the head is free	May damage hair, particularly permed or coloured hair
Ensures privacy of the client	Lacks privacy if communal
Inexpensive to run but may be less profitable as only one client can be treated	Expensive to run but may be more profitable as many clients may be treated at one time
Comfortable for most clients	Less comfortable for the older, less mobile clients or those with sensitive skins

Spa Baths

These refer to baths for sitting in rather than swimming. They vary in size and construction, from preformed, reinforced acrylic shells to block-built and tiled baths. Spa baths contain a quantity of water which is heated, chemically treated and filtered. Hydrojet circulation and air induction bubbles may also be included.

A spa bath is not drained, cleaned and refilled after each individual user. Cleaning and water change is only carried out after a specific number of people have used the bath. The frequency of water change will depend on the capacity of the bath and the number of users.

Spas may be classified into residential spas or commercial spas. Residential spas are installed for private use in the home, while commercial spas are installed for general use in premises such as hotels, health clubs, sports centres, gymnasia, salons and clinics.

Installation of spas

Spas must be installed by experienced contractors in accordance with the Swimming Pool and Allied Trades Association (SPATA) standards. The spa must be installed on a level, solid base; if the spa is to be installed on a suspended floor, consideration must be given to the weight of the bath plus water and bathers. The contractor must ensure that the support is adequate.

All spa equipment must be properly installed and connected; all components must be accessible for maintenance. The spa must be positioned so that any noise will not cause undue disturbance. Ventilation in the area of the spa should be adequate to prevent condensation.

All surfaces must be smooth, with rounded moulded edges. Uneven surfaces or sharp edges may cause accidents and injuries. The wet floor area around the spa should have a non-porous, non-slip, even surface, and must be easy to clean and sanitize. There must be adequate drainage to ensure that water spillage flows away quickly.

The contractor must ensure that the water provided to fill the spa is of satisfactory quality. If the water supply does not meet the required standards, steps must be taken to bring the water within chemical, physical and biological standards.

The contractor must advise and instruct the operator on the operational procedures required and the treatments necessary to maintain water quality and to achieve the highest standards of hygiene and safety. Advice must also be given on the correct handling and safe storage of chemicals. A manual listing all these instructions must be provided by the manufacturer or constructor and explained to the operator. The contractor must also supply a water testing kit and explain its use and limitations.

Guidelines for water standards

The source of water for the spa pool is usually from the main supply. If this is not available, water may be obtained from other sources which must be assessed and deemed suitable by a public analyst. After treatment the water should be within the following standards:

- Disinfectant levels: a bromine residual of 4–6 mg/litre for commercial spas, 2–4 mg/litre for residential spas.

- A free chlorine residual of 3–5 mg/litre for commercial spas, 1.5–3 mg/litre for residential spas. Ozone may be used in conjunction with bromine and chlorine.

- pH levels: 7.2–7.8.
- Total alkalinity: 80–160 mg/litre as calcium carbonate.
- Calcium hardness: 75–500 mg/litre as calcium carbonate.
- Total dissolved solids: less than 1500 mg/litre.

Proper standards of disinfection must be maintained at all times. The environmental health officer for the local authority will carry out a routine assessment of the biological purity of the spa water. The recommendation for spa water is as follows:

- To contain less than 100 bacteria per ml capable of growing on agar in two days at 37 °C.
- To be free from coliforms, pseudomonas, staphylococcus and faecal streptococcus in 100 ml water.

Purification

Organic and nitrogenous impurities are introduced into the spa water during normal use, therefore filtration and chemical treatment is essential to remove and break down this matter and to purify the recycled water. Algae growths may occur in some spas, and while these are not generally harmful to health, they make surfaces slippery and make the water look unattractive. A number of spa disinfectants are effective in limiting these growths, but if necessary, recommended algicides may be used. Foaming may occur as a result of soap being introduced into the spa after users have showered. This can be removed using an anti-foam agent.

Additional chemicals

In addition to the chemicals discussed above, other chemical products may be required to maintain water standards as listed below:

1 Aluminium sulphate – to aid filtration.
2 Calcium chloride – to raise calcium hardness.
3 Polyelectrolyte products – to aid filtration.
4 Sodium bicarbonate – to raise total alkalinity.
5 Sodium carbonate (soda ash) – to raise pH.
6 Sodium hydrogen sulphate – to lower pH.
7 Sodium thiosulphate – to dechlorinate and debrominate water.
8 Sequestering agents – to protect against staining and scale formation.

Use of spa pools

1 To promote relaxation.
2 To relieve muscular aches and pains.
3 To ease joint pain and stiffness.

Effects

1 An increase in the circulation.
2 An increase in heart/pulse rate.
3 A fall in blood pressure as the superficial blood vessels dilate.
4 A rise in body temperature.
5 The warmth induces muscle relaxation.
6 Soothing of sensory nerve endings.

7   An increase in cell metabolism due to warmth and increased circulation.

8   Increased pressure near the jets has an invigorating effect.

Contraindications

These should be displayed near the pool and must be explained to each client. Clients must seek medical advice before using the spa if any of the following conditions apply:

1   Heart disease or circulatory conditions such as high or low blood pressure.

2   A history of thrombosis, embolism or phlebitis.

3   Pregnancy.

4   Chest conditions such as asthma and bronchitis.

5   Epilepsy or diabetes.

6   Undiagnosed swellings.

7   If taking medication.

8   Following recent operation.

Do not use the spa if you are suffering any of the following:

- Headache, migraine, faintness, dizziness, fever.

- Any infections such as colds, flu, etc.

- Skin diseases or infections.

- Extensive bruising or any history of haemorrhage.

- Cuts and abrasions.

- Athlete's foot or verruca.

- After eating a meal or drinking alcohol.

- If on a low calorie diet.

Dangers in the use of spa pools

1   Nausea, faintness, dizziness or headache may result from overuse. Limit the time spent in the spa to 10–20 minutes.

2   Cross infection of micro-organisms.

3   Skin irritation caused by the chemicals in the water.

4   Slipping or falling if the pool surround is wet and slippery.

Precautions

1   Tell the person in charge if you are to be alone in the bath.

2   Children must not use the bath without supervision.

3   Shower before and after using the bath.

4   Do not stay in the bath for too long: 10–20 minutes only.

5   Come out if feeling too hot, faint, nauseous or dizzy.

6   Enter the bath and exit slowly holding on to the safety rail.

7   Do not enter the bath if it already contains the recommended number of bathers.

8   Check the spa temperature before use, the maximum safe temperature is 40 °C (104 °F).

9   Do not sit directly in front of the jets.

10   Shower after bathing, to cool down.

Figure 11.4 A spa pool

Operation and care of spas

Those responsible for the operation and care of spa pools must be familiar with and operate according to the legislation and codes of practice related to spa pools. Copies of these documents should be available at all times and studied in detail. These include:

1 Health and Safety at Work Act 1974.
2 Safety in Swimming Pools – Health and Safety Commission and Sports Council.
3 The Swimming Pool and Allied Trades Association (SPATA) Guidelines.

4 Code of Practice for Hygiene in Beauty Salons and Clinics.

The highest standards of hygiene and safety must be practised at all times. Every precaution must be taken to avoid cross infection or injury to the client.

Operator responsibilities

Spa baths differ in size, construction and in mode of operation. It is therefore important that each operator is fully conversant with all the details in the manufacturer's instruction manual for their particular spa. This must be obtained from the manufacturer or contractor when the bath is installed. It is the contractor's duty to explain and discuss the procedures with the operator and to give advice as required.

> As a supervisor, you have a legal responsibility under the health and safety legislation to ensure the safety of every client. Make sure that you have followed all the guidelines for operating the bath.

The operator must carry out the following procedures in accordance with the manufacturer's instructions:

1 Fill the bath to the correct level with water and ensure that this level is maintained.

2 Ensure that the pump, filter and any other devices are working correctly and are regularly cleaned and maintained.

3 Maintain the correct disinfection levels in the bath at all times; chlorine or bromine are generally added to the water either manually or automatically. It is recommended that a bromine residual of 4–6 mg/litre should be maintained in the water of a commercial spa or a chlorine residual of 3–5 mg/litre. Excess of these chemicals may cause skin irritation and smarting of the eyes.

4 Maintain the correct pH levels in the bath at all times: 7.2–7.8 is the recommended range, 7.4–7.6 is the ideal. The correct pH level is important to prevent corrosion and scale formation, and for effective disinfection and client comfort. All commercial spas should have automatic controllers to provide continuous monitoring and control of disinfectant and pH levels.

5 Clean the waterline regularly with the recommended non-foaming cleaner. This improves the hygiene standards and the appearance of the bath.

6 Remove any foam which may occur with an anti-foaming agent as this affects the clarity of the water.

7 Add a sequestering agent at the first sign of staining or scale formation which will be unattractive and may cause corrosion and block pipework.

8 Maintain a water temperature of 38 °C. The water temperature must not exceed the maximum recommended temperature of 40 °C.

9 Change the water and clean the bath and its equipment regularly. The frequency of this operation will depend on the size and usage of the bath. A daily change may be required for heavily used commercial baths. The current guideline indicates that the water should be changed when the number of users has equalled one half of the spa water capacity; for example, for a bath containing 660 gallons of water, 330 bathers may use the bath before a change of water is required. Clean the bath with a recommended cleaning agent before refilling.

Chemicals must not be mixed with each other, either in a dry state or in solution. All chemicals must be added to the spa water as indicated in the instruction manual, either directly or via a chemical feeder.

10 Test the chemical levels regularly according to the manufacturer's instructions.

11 Record all tests, changes and any maintenance work undertaken. For every chemical test, the time, result and action taken must be recorded in a record book or chart. This must be accessible to all operators. An instrument to continuously record disinfectant and pH levels is strongly recommended.

12 Keep detailed client records, which should include usage of the bath.

13 Ensure that bathers are seated correctly in the pool. They must be observed at all times, and, should they become unwell, assist them carefully out of the pool.

14 Ensure that the number of bathers in the pool at any one time does not exceed the number recommended for that pool.

15 Rowdy behaviour must not be allowed in the spa. Such behaviour must be dealt with quickly and politely but firmly. All those involved should be asked to refrain from such behaviour or told to leave the pool. Help should be sought from colleagues, supervisors or managers if the situation becomes difficult.

16 Take particular care with the handling and storage of chemicals. Read and follow guidelines on the packages. Be aware of the legislative requirements regarding these products.

17 Operators must be up to date with any new guidelines and legislative requirements relating to spa pools and chemical products.

Protection of the operator

For the protection and safety of the operator, the following protective clothing should be worn when handling chemicals: This is a legal requirement

- Apron: a bib-type apron in PVC.
- Gloves: waterproof.
- Goggles: chemical BSI standard.
- Respirator mask: recommended type.
- A first aid box with an eyewash bottle should be kept near the spa bath.

Preparation of the client

1 Greet client in a pleasant manner and reassure her.

2 Complete a record card.

3 Check for contraindications and explain these to the client. Seek medical advice where there is uncertainty.

4 Conduct the client to the changing room and explain the procedure.

5 Give the client a robe and towel.

6 Ask the client to remove jewellery, glasses and contact lenses, change into a swimsuit and cover the hair if desired.

7 Explain the importance of taking a shower before entering the bath, for reasons of hygiene, and to remove any oils, lotions, make-up or perfume.

Ask the client to rinse thoroughly to remove all traces of soap as any residue may affect the chemical balance of the water and produce foaming if carried into the bath.

8   Conduct the client to the bath and show her where to enter.

9   Advise the client to sit between the jets.

10 Tell the client that the recommended time in the bath is 10–20 minutes (maximum time is 20 minutes). The client should come out immediately if she feels unwell, dizzy or weak.

11 Observe the spa at all times when in use, give assistance as required.

12 Explain the importance of taking a shower after the bath to cool down and wash off any residue.

13 Advise the client to dry thoroughly and moisturize the skin. The client should then rest or receive further treatment such as massage.

Paraffin Wax to the Hands and Feet

Paraffin wax treatment is usually used for the hands and feet but can be used for the face and body.

Figure 11.5   A paraffin wax heater

Equipment

When cold, the wax is whitish and solid, but when heated it liquefies and clarifies. Wax is heated in containers, which vary in size and shape. The larger models have a water jacket and automatic temperature controls. Wax is heated and maintained at a temperature of 45–49 °C. The warm wax is applied in layers using a brush or ladle; when treating hands and feet these can be quickly dipped into the wax. Each layer of wax is allowed to dry and become white before the next coat is applied. A build up of six coats is desirable. The area is then wrapped in polythene, greaseproof paper or tinfoil and covered with a towel to retain the heat. The application of wax can be messy and care must be taken to cover the floor and clothing before the treatment starts.

Uses

1   To relieve pain.

2   To promote relaxation.

3   To soften the skin and cuticles.

4   To increase the circulation.

5 To improve the condition of stiff, arthritic joints. Exercises given after wax may result in increased mobility.

Effects

1 The heat raises the temperature of the area.

2 There is an increase in circulation due to vasodilation, giving hyperaemia and erythema.

3 The heat induces muscle relaxation.

4 The heat soothes sensory nerve endings.

5 The stimulation of sweat glands and more sweat is produced.

6 The stimulation of sebaceous glands thus softening the skin.

7 The moisture/grease in the wax softens the skin and cuticles.

8 An increase in the metabolic rate.

Contraindications

1 Skin diseases and disorders, particularly verrucae, athlete's foot and eczema.

2 Cuts and abrasions; small cuts can be covered with a waterproof plaster.

3 Severe bruising or swelling.

4 Any infected areas of cuticle, nails or skin.

5 Undiagnosed painful areas; seek medical advice.

6 Very hairy areas.

Dangers

Burns of the skin if the temperature is too high: 49 °C is the correct temperature. (Use a sugar thermometer if the wax bath is not automatically controlled.)

Precautions

1 Cover all areas not receiving treatment.

2 Test the wax on yourself before treatment.

3 Do not hold the part in the wax bath.

Treatment technique

Preparation of the client

1 Place the client in a well-supported, comfortable sitting position.

2 Check that all jewellery has been removed.

3 Check for contraindications.

4 Cover the floor and protect the client's clothing.

5 Wash the area thoroughly with warm, soapy water, rinse and dry.

6 Explain the procedure to the client.

Procedure

1 Check the temperature of the wax on yourself and on the client.

2 Hold the part above the bath and apply a thin coat of wax with a brush or ladle and allow the wax to dry. Repeat five or six times until the part is well covered. Work quickly.

3 Cover with polythene, greaseproof paper or tinfoil and then wrap in a towel.

4 Leave the wax on for around 20 minutes.

5 Remove the towel and paper and slide off the wax.

6 Pat the area with a tissue to dry.

7 Dispose of wax into a bin.

8 Follow with other treatments.

Paraffin Wax to the Body

Wax can be applied to the body for the same uses and effects. It is messy and difficult to apply and generally requires an area or room devoted entirely to wax treatments. The therapist must work quickly and deftly to apply a good, even coating, as the wax can cool quickly when applied to large areas.

Treatment technique

1 Prepare the bed.

2 Cover with large bath towels or a blanket.

3 Cover this with a large polythene sheet.

Preparation of the client

1 The client must shower and dry thoroughly.

2 Check that all jewellery has been removed.

3 Check for contraindications.

4 Position the client on one side on the bed.

5 Protect the pubic region and gluteal fold with large tissue.

6 Explain the procedure to the client.

Procedure

1 Using a large wax bath containing hot wax at 49 °C, paint the client's back with wax. Use a wide brush and work quickly; cover the back and legs with several layers.

2 Turn the client on to her back and paint her front with wax in the same way.

3 Wrap the client in the polythene sheet and then the towel.

4 Leave the client to rest for 20 minutes. (A heat lamp can be used to maintain the heating effect if required.)

5 Unwrap the client and remove the wax from the front; turn the client and remove wax from her back.

6 Follow with a warm shower and other treatments, such as massage.

Paraffin Wax to the Face

Paraffin wax may be applied to the face as part of a facial routine. Great care must be taken in its application, avoiding the eyes, nostrils and mouth.

Uses

1 To improve the condition of dry, dehydrated, coarse skin.

2 To stimulate the secretions of sebaceous glands.

3 To improve the condition of mature, ageing skin.

4 To stimulate and cleanse a sluggish skin and remove build up of sebum and dry keratinized cells.

5 To aid the relaxation of facial muscles.

Effects

1 The heat raises the temperature of the area.

2 There is an increase in circulation due to vasodilatation, giving hyper-aemia and erythema.

3 The stimulation of sebaceous glands; this releases blockages on a sluggish skin and helps to lubricate the dry, mature skin.

4 An increase in activity of sweat glands.

5 The moisture/grease in the wax will soften the skin.

6 There is an increase in the metabolic rate, which will improve the condition of the skin.

7 The heat soothes sensory nerve endings.

8 The heat induces muscle relaxation.

Contraindications

1 Any skin disorders or diseases.

2 Skin infections (e.g. pustular acne).

3 Highly vascular, florid, couperose skins or with telangiectasis.

4 Weathered skin with windburn or sunburn.

5 Low tolerance to heat.

6 Claustrophobic or highly tense, nervous clients.

7 Cuts and abrasions of the skin(e.g. chapped skin).

Dangers

1 Burning if the temperature of the wax is too high; maintain the heat at 45–49 °C. Always test on yourself and on the client before treatment.

2 Spillages of very hot wax; do not move heated baths.

3 Igniting the wax if near a naked flame or hotplate.

Precautions

1 Test the temperature of the wax with a sugar thermometer and test on yourself.

2 Place the wax containers on a stable base away from any flame or hotplates.

3 Check for contraindications.

4 Explain the treatment to the client.

Treatment technique

Preparation of the client

1 Place the client in a well-supported, comfortable position.

2 Check that all jewellery has been removed.

3 Check for contraindications.

4 Explain the treatment to the client.

5 Cleanse the skin.

6 Cover the hair with a towel or band to the hairline.

7 Protect clothing with towels.

8 Place eye pads over the eyes.

Procedure

1 Place the wax bath on a suitable stable base near the plinth.

2 Protect the working area; cover the floor, plinth and trolley.

3 Check the temperature of the wax on a thermometer (45–49 °C), then test it on yourself (the inner wrist is a good area), then test it on the client's neck.

4 Apply the wax quickly to the face and neck using a small brush (1/2 or 1 inch); continue until a good, even coating has been applied all over (approximately six layers deep; avoid the eyes, nostrils and mouth).

5 Cover the waxed area with polythene or greaseproof paper and then a towel; again avoid the eyes, nostrils and mouth.

6 Leave the client to rest for approximately 20 minutes depending on the skin condition and desired result.

7 Maintain verbal contact throughout; the client should avoid facial movement and so instruct her to lift her hand if she is uncomfortable or in need of assistance or give her a bell to ring.

8 Remove the wax mask; it should lift off easily if the layers are thick enough.

9 Wipe the skin with tissue.

10 Extract comedones if necessary.

11 Cleanse the skin and follow with a facial routine.

REMEMBER! Feedback and after care.

Care and maintenance of wax

- Wax is supplied as large blocks; these should be covered and kept in a dry cupboard.

- Check the blocks before placing them in the bath, remove any dirt, hairs, etc. After use the wax may be disposed of by wrapping in paper and placing in a bin. Under the new Health and Safety at Work regulations the wax must be disposed of after each client.

SUMMARY

Steam treatment

Steam may be applied using steam baths or steam rooms or using facial steamers. Water is heated forming steam-humidity at 95 per cent.

Steam baths
- Steam bath: wet heat.
- Temperature: 50–55 °C.
- Treatment time: 15–20 minutes.

Dangers
1 Overheating causing fainting and dizziness.
2 Burns from touching the metal trough.
3 Cross infection of micro-organisms, as these baths are ideal breeding grounds.

Facial steamers
- Facial steamers: heating with high humidity; water in container is heated and steam delivered to face; some include ozone in treatment.
- Distance from face: 38 cm/15 inches.
- Treatment time: 5–20 minutes.
- Treatment time with ozone: 5 minutes only at distance of 46 cm/18 inches

Sauna
- Sauna: dry heat.
- Temperature: 60–80 °C building up to 110 °C as the tolerance increases.
- Humidity range: increased by applying water to coals.
- Cooler on lower shelf, hotter on upper shelf.
- Treatment time: 5–20 minutes.

Dangers
1 Fainting or dizziness.
2 Dehydration.
3 Dryness and irritation of mucous membranes.

Paraffin wax
- Paraffin wax: may be used on the face, body, hands or feet.

summary continues overleaf

summary continued from previous page

- Temperature of wax: 45–49 °C.
- Treatment time: 20–30 minutes.

Feedback

Examine the area and ask appropriate questions to obtain feedback; this will indicate if the treatment is effective, suitable and if the client is happy.

After care

Give advice on immediate after care and the routine to follow before the next treatment.

Questions

1   List three methods of applying general heat to the body and three methods of applying local heat.

2   Explain why hyperaemia and erythema occur as a result of heat on the tissues.

3   State what happens to the following when the body is heated:
(a) The heart and pulse rate.
(b) The blood pressure.

4   Explain why there is an increase in the activity of sweat glands during heat treatments.

5   List the four factors which influence the extent of the effects when giving heat treatments.

6   Give six advantages of using a steam bath rather than steam room.

7   Give the temperatures recommended for the following treatments:
(a) Steam bath.
(b) Sauna.
(c) Wax application.

8   Explain briefly why the following conditions are contraindications to heat treatment:
(a) Heart and circulatory conditions.
(b) Thrombosis.
(c) Faintness.
(d) Diabetes.

9   Give three dangers associated with sauna treatments.

questions continues overleaf

questions continued from previous page

10 Explain the procedure for preparing the sauna and the client before sauna treatment.

11 The facial steamer may be used for steam only or may include ozone. Give the timing and distance for treatment when using:
   (a) Steam only.
   (b) Steam with ozone.

12 List five contraindications to facial steam treatment.

13 Explain the precautions to be taken before the application of wax treatments.

14 Describe the care and maintenance of paraffin wax.

Oral questions

Facial steamers

1 (a) How would your client benefit from facial steam treatment?
   (b) What skin types would benefit from this treatment and why?

2 Are there any skin types that would be unsuitable for this treatment?

3 Why is it important to use distilled water in the tank?

4 How long prior to treatment would you turn the steamer on?

5 Some steamers produce ozone as well as steam; would you take any precautions if using this type of equipment?

6 How would you ensure the safety of the client?

7 What would your procedure be after the treatment?

8 What timing and distances would you select for the following:

Skin types	Timing	Distance
Greasy/seborrhoeic		
Normal skin		
Dry skin		

Steam baths

1 Explain how you prepare the steam bath/cabinet.

2 Explain how you would prepare the client.

3 (a) What temperature should the bath reach?
   (b) What would be the humidity?

4 How long would the client remain in the bath?

5 What is the procedure after treatment?

questions continues overleaf

questions continued from previous page

Sauna baths – dry heat

1   How would you choose between steam and sauna as a preheating treatment?
2   What reasons are there for using steam and sauna treatments?
3   Why is the heat in the sauna dry heat?
4   Where would you advise the client to sit on the first treatment and why?
5   What should the temperature range and humidity be?
6   How would you prevent cross infection?
7   What is the treatment time?

Spas

1   Where does the water for spa pools come from?
2   How is the water maintained and purified?
3   How would you explain the procedure to the client?
4   What is the maximum safe temperature for a bath?
5   What dangers must you be aware of to ensure safety of your client?
6   What is the ideal pH level in the bath?
7   Why is the correct pH level important?
8   The waterline becomes dirty over time, how do you deal with this?
9   What advice would you give the client following a spa bath?

Paraffin wax treatments

1   Explain the benefits of wax treatments.
2   When would you not recommend wax treatment?
3   What are the two main dangers of wax treatments?
4   At what temperature should the wax be maintained?
5   What areas of the body are suitable for wax treatment?
6   How does the wax produce beneficial effects?
7   How should wax be disposed of?

Case Studies

Student therapists often find case studies quite daunting but like any assessment they are an opportunity to demonstrate your knowledge. If you do not feel confident in your knowledge, than equip yourself with a good textbook which contains the information you require.

Each case study will provide a scenario, **read this very carefully**.

Write a list of the relevant points which will provide you with the basis for selecting the treatments. This list will include:

1 **Age:** this will have some effect on your choice of treatments. Some treatments will be more suitable for the mature client while other treatments will be more suitable for the younger client.

2 **Lifestyle details:** these are very important because they will also influence the choice of treatment. They will offer guidance regarding the timing and length of treatment. The client must be able and happy to attend the salon at the appointed times. She must agree with the plan and the cost. Explain why this is an important factor. Is the client working, is she stressed? these factors will point to the more relaxing treatments; or does she lead a leisurely life with sufficient time for longer treatments? You may be provided with other

details; include and use all the facts that are presented to you. Discuss each detail and explain how and why they influenced the choice of treatment and the after care advice.

3 **Details of her condition:** this will be the basis of your treatment selection. You must always choose what, in your opinion, is the best possible treatment for the client. You must be able to justify and discuss your decision, giving the advantages and limitations. Explain how you would guide and explain the treatment to the client taking into account her needs and requests. Consider health, safety and hygiene issues, outline how you maintained safe practice and ensured the comfort of the client.

- For a facial condition, explain the preparation of the face, cleansing, toning, skin analysis, contraindications, any pre-treatment, details of how you performed the treatment, the precautions you took, the contra-actions you were watching for, the feedback you obtained and the after care advice you gave.

- For a body condition, explain the examination of posture, the testing of muscle tone, the observation of type and distribution of fat, the checking for fluid retention, the examination of the skin, the checking for contraindications. The procedure will be similar to that for a facial condition.

4 **The client's past experience of salon treatment:** were the past treatments successful? Was the experience positive and enjoyable? What were her likes and dislikes and what are the client's expectations?

All these factors will also influence your decisions.

You may be offered guidance within the question regarding the content to be included. Read this carefully and provide as much detail as you can and feel is required. Analyze the problem; discuss and give reasons for your choices; justify your decisions; evaluate the effectiveness and limitations of the treatment.

Refer to health, safety and hygiene issues throughout.

Glossary

Blood pressure The pressure exerted against the artery walls, during contraction of the heart (systolic pressure) and relaxation of the heart (diastolic pressure). Normal blood pressure is around 120 (systolic)/80 (diastolic).

Connectors or inter-neurones These connect one neurone with another.

Couperosed skin A redness of the skin.

Desquamation A flaking or erosion of the surface layer of the statum corneum of the skin.

Diaphorectic effect An increase in the production of sweat.

Electrolyte A chemical compound which dissociates into ions and carries a current.

Erythema A reddening of the skin; this happens as a result of vasodilation.

Heart rate The rate at which the heart beats; this is the same as the pulse rate.

Hyperaemia An increase in blood flow to an area.

Metabolic rate The rate of chemical reaction in body cells.

Metabolites Waste products of metabolism.

Motor nerves or neurones These nerves transmit impulses from brain and spinal cord to muscles and glands.

Occlude To stop or obstruct.

Oedema or edema Swelling of an area due to excess fluid.

Phlebitis Inflammation of a vein.

Sebaceous glands Glands in the skin which secrete a fatty substance called sebum.

Seborrhoea Excessive secretion of sebum from sebaceous glands.

Sensory nerves or neurones These nerves transmit impulses from sensory organs, such as skin, eyes and ears, to the spinal cord and brain.

Stasis An area of stagnation due to poor circulation.

Telangiectasis Small, red spots on the skin caused by dilated capillaries.

Tension nodules Areas within a muscle where muscle fibres show increase in tone.

Thrombosis The formation of a blood clot in blood vessels.

Vasoconstriction Constriction of blood vessels (i.e. the lumen get smaller).

Vasodilation Dilation of blood vessels (i.e. the lumen of the blood vessels get larger).

Bibliography

Bennett, Ruth, *The Science of Beauty Therapy* (Hodder & Stoughton, 1992).

Gray, H., *Gray's Anatomy* (Churchill Livingstone, 1980).

Freemantle, Michael, *Chemistry in Action* (Macmillan, 1987).

Forster, Angela and Palastanga, Nigel, *Clayton's Electrotherapy* (Bailliere Tindall, 1985).

Hutchinson Encyclopedia (Guild Publishing London, 1988).

Kahn, Joseph, *Principles and Practice of Electrotherapy* (Churchill Livingstone, 1987).

Peberdy, W. G., *Sterilisation and Hygiene in the Beauty Professions* (1987).

Ross, J. S. and Wilson K. J. W., *Anatomy and Physiology* (Churchill Livingstone, 1988).

Simmons, John, *The Beauty Salon and Its Equipment* (Macmillan, 1989).

Answers

Oral questions

Direct high frequency

1 High frequency alternating current.

2 ■ The ozone produced has a drying effect.
  ■ Sebaceous glands are stimulated, releasing blockages.
  ■ Heat is produced in the tissues increasing the metabolic rate of the cells which promotes healing and improves the condition of the skin.
  ■ Sparking destroys bacteria and promotes the healing of pustules and papules.

3 The treatment destroys bacteria.

4 The ozone and the ultraviolet produced destroys bacteria.

5 Jewellery is metal and will conduct electricity.

6 It can be recommended because it increases sebaceous secretions but the treatment should be for 4–5 minutes only.

7 Alcohol is highly inflammable.

8 No more than 7 mm or ¼ inch away from the tissues.

9 The ozone produced destroys bacteria. Ultraviolet rays produced in the gap are also destructive to the tissues.

10 The therapist's hand should either hold the machine cable away from the client or be placed on the pillow, away from the client's head.

11 ■ Ask the client how the treatment felt, was she comfortable, relaxed, happy during treatment?
   ■ How did the skin feel?
   ■ Examine the skin reaction. Was there a good even glow or was it very red, showing sensitivity?

12 Wash the electrode with warm soapy water and wipe with disinfectant but make sure not to wet the metal contact.

13 Small powder particles can be inhaled and cause respiratory problems.

Indirect high frequency

1 It is a current that alternates rapidly.

2 Because the current is not applied directly to the area through an electrode. The current is applied via a saturator held in the hand and the therapist draws off the current through her hands as they massage the face. The therapist is part of the circuit around which the current flows.

3 ■ Sebaceous glands are stimulated to produce more sebum.

- Increased circulation and warmth created increases the metabolic rate of the cells thus improving the condition of the skin.
- The cream used has a lubricating effect.

4 It refers to chemical reactions that take place in the cells when the cells use up nutrients and eliminate waste products more quickly.

5 The client would experience a slight shock.

6 Because of its lubricating effect which is beneficial for dry, dehydrated, lined skin.
It provides a good medium and reduces friction as the hands move over the part.
It promotes a soothing treatment.

7 Talc is sometimes indicated for a superficial stimulating effect. Great care must be taken; use only a small amount of talc and apply it carefully and gently to the face. The powder particles if inhaled are a hazard and there is a risk of causing respiratory problems.

8 Treat for approximately 5–20 minutes depending on the reaction of the skin and tolerance of the client.

9 If there were any contra-actions I would stop immediately, e.g.
1 Rash or redness of the skin caused by over treating.
2 Allergic reaction to the cream.
3 Faintness.
4 Nausea.
5 Restlessness.

10 To ensure the client is holding the saturator in the hand without jewellery and that she continues to hold it firmly throughout treatment.

Mechanical massage

1 The manipulations are deeper and effects greater.

2 Very effective on large bulky areas, less tiring than manual massage.

3 Treatment rather impersonal and sometimes not as pleasing to the client.

4 - The heavier heads will provide a more thorough, deeper treatment and produce better and more effective results.
- The increased circulation to the area and the continuous heavy pressure on adipose tissue may aid the dispersal of fatty deposits if the client is on a reducing diet.

5 To adapt to body contours.
- The curved sponge head is used on legs and is similar to effleurage.
- The hard rubber heads are similar to petrissage.
- Spiky heads are similar to percussion.

6 - Areas of fatty deposits and areas of cellulite – as the increased circulation will improve metabolic rate in the tissues and aid the dispersal of fatty deposits, providing the client is on a reducing diet.
- Clients with poor circulation; the flow of blood in the veins is speeded up removing deoxygenated blood and waste products. The arterial circulation is

increased, bringing oxygen and nutrients to the area.

- Clients with dry flaky skin; the friction of the heads on the skin will have a desquamating effect which will improve the texture of the skin.

7 - Yes, broken/dilated capillaries or bruising.
- Internal organs could be damaged if pressure was too heavy and treatment too vigorous on the abdomen.

8 - Taking care to feed the tissues onto the head.
- Avoid repeatedly working over the same area (keep the head moving).
- Make sure the head is parallel with the surface.
- Adapt pressure to suit the tissues.

9 - Increase in circulation, improving condition of tissues.
- Increase in metabolic rate, improving the condition of tissues.
- Rise in temperature which promotes healing and relaxation.
- Erythema improves skin colour.
- Friction of the head aids desquamation.

10 It is a safety factor, in case the head flies off hitting the client or anyone else.

11 Because oil causes deterioration of the sponge head.

12 - Washed my hands, then cleaned the part.
- Placed sponge heads in clean disposable plastic bags or washable covers.

- Washed rubber heads in soapy water.

13 On well-toned clients with areas requiring desquamation.

Facial vacuum suction treatments

1 Because air has been sucked out of the cup creating a vacuum.

2 By turning the intensity control up and down.

3 To fill less than 20 per cent of the cup.

4 - For general cleansing of the skin – it helps to loosen blockages and comedones, thus cleansing the pores. It aids removal of dead keratinized cells, improving the texture of the skin.
- Deep cleansing of greasy seborrhoeic skin – as above, particularly the desquamating effect, as greasy skins become dull and sallow due to the excess sebum on the skin which delays the rate of the desquamating process.
- Speeds up the removal of waste products via the lymphatic system and increases the circulation which will improve the tone and condition of the skin.
- To stimulate and improve dry, dehydrated skin – the increase in circulation will help to balance the moisture content. The desquamating effect will improve the texture of the skin and the oil will help to lubricate the skin.

5 Working towards the nearest set of lymph nodes.

6 - Superficial and deep cervical.
- Anterior auricular (parotid).

- Post auricular (mastoid).
- Submandibular.
- Submental.

7
- By removing my finger from the hole.
- By depressing the flesh.

8
- To avoid overstretching the skin.
- To avoid causing broken capillaries.

9 Perpendicular to the skin and fill only 20 per cent.

10 Wash in hot water and detergent, then soak in disinfectant such as Milton.

11 10–12 minutes depending on skin reaction.

12
- Remove the oil.
- Examine the skin and note any adverse reaction.
- Ask the client if she had been comfortable throughout and if she had relaxed and enjoyed the treatment.
- Ask if the client was satisfied?

Body vacuum suction treatments

1
- Using a single ventouse which is manually moved over the part.
- Using multiple pulsating cups. This enables the therapist to carry out other treatments on the client (e.g. a mini manicure, file and polish, eyebrow shape).

2
- On soft fatty deposits of the body.
- Areas of cellulite.
- To aid non-systemic oedema and areas of fluid retention.

3 (a) Yes, poor technique may cause broken capillaries, bruising, or stretching the skin.

(b) By making sure that:
- The pressure isn't too high.
- The vacuum is released before lifting the cup off.
- When lifting and gliding do not push the cup down – lift and glide.

4
- By working with the contours of the body in sweeping lines.
- Overlapping the previous stroke by ½ inch or 1 cm.

5 The cup size must fit the part, to form a seal, and be large enough to be effective.

6
- After covering the area approximately six times and producing a good, even erythema.
- If there were any contra-actions stop immediately.

7
- Preheat the area. This could be followed by mechanical or manual massage to increase circulation.
- Followed by vacuum suction.
- Followed by EMS or galvanic. This would be the order of treatment, any two or three could be selected depending on the needs of the client.

8 No. The areas under the pads will have become very sensitive during galvanic treatment and further treatments should not be given.

Facial galvanic treatment:

Disincrustation

1 Direct current sometimes referred to as constant current. It flows in one direction only.

2 ■ Careful skin analysis.
■ Skin sensitivity test (hot and cold, sharp and soft).

3 Because the treatment has a drying effect on the skin and is not suitable for mature, dry, dehydrated skin. It can be used for a short time 4–5 minutes for its stimulating effects but there are better treatments (e.g. iontophoresis).

4 To make sure that the client can feel hot and cold, sharp and soft.

5 If she had suffered any nerve damage such as Bell's palsy, stroke, Parkinson's disease or nerve injury, as the sensory nerve endings may not register sensations of touch, heat or pain and the nerves would not transmit stimuli to the brain.

6 I would not proceed with disincrustation or any other galvanic or heat treatment.
  I would carefully explain the reasons to the client and offer another suitable treatment.

7 ■ For general cleansing treatment for combination and greasy skin.
■ For deep cleansing seborrhoeic skin.
■ To stimulate a sluggish skin with a build-up of keratinized cells and comedomes.

8 Saline solution (2 teaspoons of salt stirred into 1 litre of water).

9 By means of 2 electrodes:
■ One is the cathode (−) which is the active electrode used on the face.
■ The other one is the anode (+) which is the inactive electrode,

this may be held in the hand or a plate electrode may be strapped to the arm.

10 ■ The electrodes must be covered with lint or special sponge covers.
■ The cathode cover is moistened with saline solution or product to produce its effect and help absorb the debris on the skin.
■ The cover must be changed when reversing the polarity.

11 ■ If saline solution is used at the cathode, sodium hydroxide is formed due to electrolysis of salt and water. Sodium hydroxide is an alkali which saponifies sebum (saponifies – breaks down the sebum to a soapy liquid). It also breaks down the keratin in skin cells. Products produce the same results.
■ Fluid is drawn to the cathode, softening the area.
■ The irritation produced by the current results in vasodilation (increased lumen of blood vessels), hyperaemia (increased blood flow to the area), erythema (reddening of the skin).
■ The skin is softened, cleaned and there is an improvement in colour and condition.

12 (a) Yes, the sodium hydroxide is an alkali and alters the pH of the skin (as it becomes more alkaline). This destroys the acid mantle thus reducing the protective function of the skin against micro-organisms.
(The acid mantle is a mixture of sebum and sweat which forms an

acidic coating on the skin pH 4.5–6).

(b) Yes, by switching the polarity at the end of the treatment. By switching the polarity on the machine, the anode becomes the active electrode, hydrochloric acid is formed at the anode which restores the acid mantle.

13 Treatment time 10–15 minutes depending on reaction of client. Reverse polarity to restore acid mantle for 2–4 minutes.

14 ▪ Test the current on self, before securing the electrodes.
▪ Place the inactive rod in the client's hand or strap a plate to the arm.
▪ Place the active electrode on a sensitive part of the face (e.g. forehead).
▪ Explain the importance of indicating when a tingling sensation is felt.
▪ Turn the current up very slowly until the client just feels it.

15 A sensitive area is where the current would feel most intense. If the current was turned up on an insensitive area, when the electrode moved to the sensitive part the intensity would be too high. This would be very uncomfortable for the client.

16 ▪ Dry skin offers a resistance to the current.
▪ When the skin becomes more moist the resistance is lowered and current intensity increases.
▪ The higher intensity will be too uncomfortable for the client.

17 It depends on the client's tolerance, the amount of current must only be as high as the client can comfortably tolerate, up to 2 mA.

18 The skin is very thin in this area and during the treatment the client may experience a 'flash' as the electrode passes near this area.

Facial galvanic treatment: Iontophoresis

1 Direct current (constant current).

2 By means of two electrodes:
▪ One will be the cathode (−), the other will be the anode (+).
▪ The active electrode may be two rollers or ball electrodes.
▪ The inactive electrode is a rod for holding in the hand or a plate which is strapped to the upper arm.

3 This depends on the product used:
▪ If the product is negatively charged the cathode must be the active electrode (anion active).
▪ If the product is positively charged the anode must be the active electrode (cation active).

4 Because like charges repel, opposite charges attract.
▪ The cathode (−) must be used to repel negative anions into the skin.
▪ The anode (+) must be used to repel positive cations into the skin.

5 A wide variety of skin conditions can be treated in this way because there are products available to improve most skin conditions. Accurate skin analysis to determine the client's needs and selection of the appropriate product is essential.

6 The main effect depends on the product used (e.g. moisturising product for dry mature skin). Other effects are due to stimulation by the direct current:
   (a) Vasodilation, hyperaemia, erythema will improve tone/colour.
   (b) Increased cell metabolism will improve condition.
   (c) Desquamation improves texture and condition.

7 Low intensity current is required which must only be as high as the client can tolerate, 0.5–2.0 mA.

8 Up to 20 minutes.

Body galvanic treatments

1 Direct current (constant current).

2 Client with areas of fat and/or cellulite, or areas with poor circulation.

3 ▪ The client is placed in a comfortable position.
   ▪ All jewellery or metal pins or studs are removed.
   ▪ Treatment is explained to the client and the importance of reporting any irritating spots, any hot spots or any discomfort.
   ▪ The area is thoroughly washed to remove sebum or any lotions or products which may have been applied to the skin.
   ▪ Skin sensitivity test is carried out.

4 By means of two plate electrodes.
   ▪ One will be the cathode (−) which will be the active electrode.
   ▪ One will be the anode (+) which will be the inactive electrode.

5 The electrodes must be evenly covered with lint or sponge covers approximately ½ inch to 1 cm thick. This is important because if there were uneven areas the current would concentrate there (current will take the path of least resistance). The pads must be thick enough to absorb any chemicals produced.

6 (a) ▪ Sodium hydroxide is formed because of electrolysis of salt and water. This softens the skin and tissues.
       ▪ Hydrogen is released which stimulates the tissues.
       ▪ Tissue fluid is drawn to the area.
       ▪ Vasodilation with hyperaemia and erythema.
       ▪ Heat is produced, this should feel even with no hot spots.
       ▪ Irritation of sensory nerves increases conductivity of nerves.

   (b) ▪ Although the anode is the inactive electrode certain effects will occur but they are not used in the treatment if salt solution is used.
       ▪ Hydrochloric acid is formed which tightens and hardens the tissues.
       ▪ Oxygen is released which increases the vitality of the tissues.
       ▪ Vasodilation with hyperaemia and erythema but not as great as under cathode.
       ▪ Has an analgesic effect as it decreases conductivity of nerves.
       ▪ Heat is produced.

7 Yes, there is:
  - An increase in circulation.
  - An increase in metabolic rate.
  - An increase in lymphatic drainage.
  - Lowering of blood pressure.

8 Because burns can be caused. These are caused by a build-up of heat or a build-up of chemicals.

Thermal burns
These are caused by a build-up of heat, a red sore patch appears which may or may not blister. These are caused if the current intensity is too high. If the current flow is too long. If there are high points of resistance such as freckles.

Chemical burns
  - Chemical burns under the cathode (−): a red sore mark changes to a grey oozing wound. It appears due to a build-up of sodium hydroxide.
  - Chemical burns under the anode (+): a red hard lump appears which changes to a dry scab, this is due to a build up of hydrochloric acid.

Make sure the client is not lying with full body weight on the pads.

9 Shock may be caused by:
  (a) Faulty equipment controls not functioning correctly, always check the machine.
  (b) If the current is increased or decreased suddenly, always turn intensity up and down very slowly.
  (c) If the skin resistance drops suddenly. As the skin becomes moist the resistance decreases, reduce current as resistance drops. Stay with the client.

10 Contact the qualified first aider to deal with this situation.

11 This must be within the tolerance of the client who must feel comfortable throughout, up to 0.5 mA per square cm of pad.

12 Up to 20 minutes.

13 The pressure on the pads from the weight of the body may cause a thermal burn.

14 When saline solution is substituted with anti-cellulite gels/ampoules that contain charged ions which are repelled into the skin using the appropriate electrode.

Facial electrical muscle stimulation (facial faradic)

1 Interrupted direct current

2 For a client with:
  (a) Poor muscle tone.
  (b) Loss of firm contours.
  (c) Slight puffiness.

3 There are three ways:
  (a) A mushroom disc electrode as the active electrode used on the face with the inactive plate electrode strapped to the arm.
  (b) Facial block (double disc electrode): this has both the active and inactive electrode contained in one applicator.
  (c) Facial mask electrode where the electrodes are embedded in a mask.

4 On the motor point of each muscle. Because it is the point of maximum excitation of the nerve and will produce the best contraction.

5 It is the point where the nerve enters the belly of the muscle.

6 ■ Just in front of the ear as this is where the facial nerve is most superficial and the muscles supplied by the nerve will be stimulated.
  ■ Or over a group of muscles.

7 ■ Yes, because all the electrodes are embedded in the mask they cannot be moved to accurately target individual muscles.
  ■ Client may feel claustrophobic.

8 (a) Digastric.
  (b) Procerus.
  (c) Raises the mandible, used in chewing.

9 ■ Cover the disc evenly.
  ■ Moisten the sponge with saline solution; make sure that the salt crystals have completely dissolved.
  ■ Check contraindications and ensure there are no open areas of skin.
  ■ Skin test, sharp/blunt.
  ■ Make sure intensity at zero then turn up slowly during the surge.
  ■ Turn down slowly then switch off.
  ■ Keep intensity within tolerance of client.
  ■ Stay within easy reach of controls at all times.

10 6–8 contractions.

11 10–20 minutes.

Body electrical muscle stimulation (body faradic)

1 Interrupted direct current.

2 By means of graphite impregnated rubber electrodes.

3 ■ To improve contours of the body for figure reshaping.

■ To improve muscle tone in flabby muscles (e.g. after childbirth).
■ To firm pectoral muscles to improve breast sag.

4 On the motor points of the muscle as this is the area of maximum excitability; some muscles have more than one motor point.

5 Three.

6 Longitudinal padding where the pads are placed one on the upper and one on the lower motor points. The current flows through the muscle and a better contraction is produced.

7 Duplicate padding.

8 It prevents individual control of each muscle. The muscle on one side of the body may be stronger than the other. Use the monophasic control and place the cathode on the weaker muscle.

9 ■ Check the contacts at the leads and terminals are secure.
  ■ Check that the intensity is high enough.
  ■ Check that the pads are damp enough.
  ■ Check the contact between pads and skin pads which must be contoured to the area.
  ■ If contractions were still poor, remove the pads and thoroughly clean the skin.
  ■ Check that the covering fat was not too deep!

10 ■ Make sure that the rest period is longer than the contraction period.
  ■ Not have the intensity too high.
  ■ Not treat for too long.

11 Heavy padding of the chest region can interfere with heart rhythm.

12 Skin offers resistance to the current, moist skin offers less resistance. When there is a break in the skin the current will concentrate here because the current seeks the path of least resistance. It will be very painful.

13 A heat treatment such as sauna, steam or hot showers, as warm muscles contract more efficiently than cold muscles. Therefore, lower intensity will produce a good contraction which is more comfortable for the client.

14 Warm muscles contract more readily than cold muscles. The skin would be moistened thus lowering its resistance to the current. Therefore lower current intensity would produce the same effect and would be more comfortable for the client.

15 ■ 30–40 minutes depending on client tolerance.
   ■ 2–3 times per week.
   ■ Over a period of 6–8 weeks.

16 Complete the chart:

Machine controls	Function	Special points
On/off switch	*Turns the current on and off*	Make sure all terminals are at zero
Surge control/ surge envelope	*Controls the length of the surge*	Muscles with poor muscle tone require a *longer* surge

(contd)

Relaxation control/rest period	Controls the length of rest period	Must be *longer* than the surge
Frequency control	Controls the number of *pulses* per second	Should be set between *40–80*

Microcurrent treatments

1 Low intensity modified direct current.

2 The client feels very little except very slight mild tingling. This is because the current is very low amperage measured in microamps: 1 microamp = 1/1000 milliamps.

3 ■ To improve condition of ageing skins.
   ■ To soften lines and wrinkles.
   ■ To improve or maintain muscle tone.
   ■ To improve contours of the face.
   ■ To improve skin colour and texture.
   ■ To reduce puffiness.
   ■ To soften scar tissue.
   ■ To promote relaxation.

4 ■ Increases circulation.
   ■ Improves lymphatic drainage.
   ■ Improves permeability of cell membranes.
   ■ Increases cell metabolism.
   ■ Increases production of ATP.
   ■ Improves synthesis of protein.
   ■ Stimulates cell renewal.
   ■ Improves ion exchange.
   ■ Stimulates myofibrils thus improving muscle tone.
   ■ Stimulates production of fibroblasts.

- Polar effects if unmodified direct current is used.

5 Selection depends on the effects required. Manufacturers offer guidance for their machines.

6 Twice weekly for 10–12 treatments. Recommend one per month for maintenance.

Infra-red and radiant heat treatments to face and body

1 As a preheating treatment to prepare the tissues for further treatment:
   - To increase circulation.
   - To aid the absorption of products.
   - To warm muscles prior to EMS because warm muscles contract more efficiently.
   - To promote relaxation.
   - Make the following treatment more effective.

2 - Both the lamps emit infra-red rays but of different wavelength.
   - Rays from infra-red lamps are non-luminous; radiant heat lamps are luminous (usually glow red).
   - Rays from radiant heat lamps are more irritating and penetrate deeper – 3 mm of tissue down to the dermis.
   - Rays from infra-red lamps are less irritating and penetrate 1 mm of skin in the epidermis.
   - Infra-red lamps take longer to reach maximum output, 10–15 minutes.
   - Radiant heat lamps heat up quickly to reach maximum output in 2 minutes.

3 - Heat is produced in the tissues producing a general rise in body temperature.
   - Increase in metabolic rate.
   - Vasodilation with hyperaemia and erythema.
   - Fall in blood pressure because vessels dilate.
   - Increase in heart rate.
   - Increased activity of sweat glands and elimination of waste.
   - Warm muscles contract more readily, aches and pains are relieved producing relaxation.
   - Mild heat has a soothing effect on sensory nerve endings.
   - Intense heat has an irritating effect on sensory nerve endings.

4 - The main one is burns. These may occur if the intensity is too high; If the lamp is too near the client; If skin sensation is defective, *always* test with hot and cold; If the client touches the lamp or if the lamp should fall on the client or bedding.
   - Shock from faulty apparatus.
   - Headache, faintness, eye damage, chill.

5 Stop the treatment immediately and deal with each problem accordingly.

6 - The surface of the lamp should be parallel with the part.
   - The intensity of the lamp: the hotter the lamp the further away from the client it should be placed.
   - The client's tolerance – ask the client if the heat is comfortable, explain to the client that it should feel mild and tell her that they must call you if it should get uncomfortably hot.

- Make sure the rays are not directed towards the eyes: use goggles or cotton wool for facial treatment.

7 60 cm (24 inches), keep the distance roughly between 45–90 cms (18–36 inches).

8 The cosine law.

9 The law of inverse squares.

10 20–30 minutes depending on the client's tolerance and the desired effect.

11 Because infra-red intensifies the reaction to ultraviolet.

12 ■ To get up slowly because blood pressure is lowered and there is a risk of fainting.
■ To drink plenty of water.
■ To rest, relax and take things easy.

Ultraviolet treatment

1 Three: UVA, UVB, UVC.

2 No, ultraviolet rays from the sun do not heat the tissues, infra-red rays from the sun heat the tissues.

3 No, ultraviolet rays from sunbeds do not heat the tissue. (A solarium contains bulbs emitting infra-red and tubes emitting ultraviolet rays.)

4 Mainly UVA; some sunbeds emit a small amount of UVB. All UVC rays are prevented from coming through the tubes by a phosphorus coating or other filters.

5 For the tanning effect to enhance appearance.

6 (a) Tonic effect, improving appetite and sleep and reducing irritability.

(b) Can be used to treat acne; the increase in circulation, drying effect, desquamation and abiotic effect improves the condition of the skin.

(c) Formation of vitamin D.

7 UVC rays; because they are abiotic they destroy micro-organisms.

8 Tanning is a protective function of the skin:
■ Melanocytes in the skin produce the brown pigment melanin.
■ UVA stimulate and darken the melanin granules in the skin.
■ UVB stimulate melanocytes to produce more melanin granules, therefore the tanning is slower but lasts longer than the tan produced by UVA.

9 Ultraviolet irradiation results in a chemical reaction which converts 7 dehydro-cholestrol in sebum into vitamin D.

10 Because it is necessary for the absorption of calcium and phosphorus which are important for the formation of teeth and bones.

11 ■ Causal factors for skin cancers.
■ Skin ageing due to cell damage and damage of elastin and collagen.
■ Polymorphic light eruption – red, hard, itchy papules and scaling.
■ Photosensitivity – painful itchy rash may be followed by pigmentation.
■ Damage to the eyes – inflammation of the cornea (keratitis) and conjunctiva (conjunctivitis).

12 ■ Instruction for use must be clearly written and displayed.

- The door to the cubicle must open from the outside; access should not be impeded; it must facilitate easy exit.
- Sunbeds must be positioned in a well-ventilated room to dissipate ozone and heat.
- Sunbed must be isolated in its own room so that all the rays are contained to protect others from irradiation.
- The sunbed must be cleaned before and after treatment.
- A special disinfecting agent from the manufacturer must be used.
- Sunbeds must be inspected regularly for electrical and mechanical safety.
- Servicing and repair must be carried out by a qualified electrician in accordance with manufacturer's instruction. Records must be kept of all servicing and repair.
- Faulty tubes must be replaced immediately.
- The running time of the sunbed must be recorded as the tubes wear out with use.
- Always replace bulbs or tubes with the exact same model as power may vary.
- Staff must be adequately trained and available to provide accurate advice and supervision.

13　Check with contraindicated list. If the drug is on the list do not treat the client with ultraviolet. If unsure seek the doctor's advice.

14　Explain to the client that due to hormonal changes, ultraviolet may produce uneven pigmentation (chloasma). Large brown areas of pigmentation may result. Explain that ultraviolet exposure is not advisable.

15　
- Carry out a consultation, check for contraindications.
- Discuss the skin type, the reaction to sunlight.
- Establish the date of previous exposure to UVL.
- Explain the procedure to the client, show them the sunbed.
- Explain the switch, timer, release button.
- Demonstrate the way to access and exit the sunbed.
- Explain the importance of calling for help if they feel unwell, faint, nauseous, dizzy, or too hot,
- Report any skin irritation.
- Ensure that the client takes a shower using unperfumed soap.
- Remove any metals and make-up.
- Explain the importance of wearing goggles, make sure these are disposable and sterile.
- Explain the importance of keeping strictly to the time set.

16　Because the products may sensitize the skin.

17　
- Clean the bed with disinfecting detergent provided by the manufacturer.
- Check that the sunbed is sound and that all facilities are in order.
- Check and set the switch and time.
- Place clean disposable floor covering for each client.
- Provide clean boiled towels.

- Provide sterile or disposable ultra-violet goggles for each client.
- Protect the client's hair particularly if it is tinted/highlighted.
- Ensure that the room has adequate lighting, is warm but not hot, and well ventilated.
- Ensure privacy of the client.

Facial steamers

1 (a)
- Steam would introduce the client to further treatment.
- The client's skin would be softened which would make any following treatment more effective.
- Steam treatment will aid the absorption of creams or lotions.
- The client would find the treatment relaxing.
- The healing of blemished, seborrhoeic, pustular skin would be speeded up.

(b)
- Greasy, seborrhoeic, pustular skin because of the healing and bacteriacidal effect of ozone.
- Dry, dehydrated skin because sebaceous glands are stimulated.
- Steam will aid the absorption of beneficial nourishing creams.
- Sluggish, thickened skin because steam will soften the keratinized cells and build-up of sebum.
- Mature skin because the heat will produce vasodilation and increased metabolic rate.

2
- Yes, highly vascular red, couperosed skin.
- Very sensitive skin.
- Very dry or weathered skin.
- Rosacea or telangiectasis.
- Abrasions or chapped skin.

3 To prevent impurities or chemicals clogging up the steamer.

4 Until vapour/steam is produced: usually 5–10 minutes.

5 Yes, if inhaled, ozone can damage the respiratory tract. Treat for 5 minutes only at a distance of 46 cm/18 inches, observe the client throughout.

6
- Ensure that the steamer is positioned safely away from the client.
- Ensure the tank is filled with distilled water.
- Switch on 5–10 minutes before the treatment.
- Help the client on to the couch and make them comfortable.
- Ask the client to remove all jewellery.
- Check for contraindications.
- Cleanse the face.
- Explain the procedure to the client.
- Cover the client's eyes with damp cotton wool pads.
- Position the steamer safely and ensure that it cannot overturn.
- Make sure there is no water spitting out.
- Stay with the client throughout.

7 When the time is up:
- Switch the steamer off and move to a safe place away from client or others.

- Dry the skin and remove eyepads.
- Extract comedones.
- Examine the skin for any reaction.
- Ask the client if they were comfortable and happy with the treatment.
- Follow with further treatment.

8 What timing would you select for the following:

Skin types	Timing	Distance
Greasy, seborrhoeic	*15–20 minutes*	*10–15 inches*
Normal skin	*10–15 minutes*	*10–15 inches*
Dry skin	*3–7 minutes*	*15–18 inches*

Steam baths

1
- Wipe over the interior of the bath with sterilizing detergent.
- Check the water tank, ensure at least 2 inches of water to cover the element.
- Place clean towels over the seat and make sure that the client is protected from contact with metal or direct steam.
- Place clean paper roll over the floor.
- Place clean towel over the aperture to prevent loss of steam.
- Switch on, set temperature and allow 15–20 minutes to heat up.

2
- The client must remove all jewellery, contact lenses, glasses.
- The client must shower prior to entering the cabinet.
- Check feet for infections or other contraindications.

- Show client how to use the bath and help her in.
- Place towel around her neck to prevent steam escaping.

3 (a) 50–55 °C
(b) 95 per cent

4 15–20 minutes.

5
- Help the client from the bath and into the shower.
- Offer the client a friction rub to aid desquamation.
- Offer them a warm place to rest for 20–30 minutes or to receive further treatments such as massage, but they must not exercise.

Sauna baths – dry heat

1 It would depend on availability and client preference. If the client suffered from claustrophobia or any respiratory problems, the steam bath would be the choice because the head is free.

2 They are very good as preheating treatments as they induce relaxation and result in deep cleansing.

3 Because the sauna is constructed of pinewood which absorbs moisture.

4 On the lower benches, as hot air rises and the upper benches are hotter. Instruct the client to come out of sauna if they begin to feel faint, dizzy, nauseous, giddy, tense or if they have any trouble breathing or with dryness in nose of lungs.

5
- Temperature = 60°–80 °C.
- Humidity = 50–70 per cent.

6
- Scrub the benches and floor thoroughly with disinfectant

specifically manufactured for use in saunas.

- Protect the floor with paper towel.
- Cover the benches with clean towels.
- Ensure that the client takes a shower before and after treatment.
- Provide paper slippers for the clients to wear.

7 This depends on the client's tolerance, begin with 5 minutes and work up to 15–20 minutes.

Spas

1 Usually from the main supply.

2 The water is continually filtered and chemicals are added to the water. A fully trained person must be in charge of maintaining water purity, they must be familiar with and operate according to the legislation and codes of practice related to spa pools.

3
- This is a heating treatment which will improve the effects of further treatments. It will stimulate the circulation and help you to relax.
- Take a shower to remove any products such as perfumes, lotions, etc.
- Be careful as you enter the bath, hold on to the rail and walk in slowly.
- Do not sit directly in front of the jets, they may cause bruising.
- Relax and remain in the bath for 10–20 minutes.
- Come out slowly and take a shower.
- Put your gown on and return to the cubicle.
- Come out immediately if you feel at all uncomfortable, feel too hot giddy or nauseous, etc.

4 40 °C or 104 °F (38 °C is the ideal temperature).

5
- Cross infection by micro-organisms from one client to another.
- Skin irritation caused by chemicals in the pool.
- Nausea, dizziness, faintness, heat exhaustion.

6 7.4–7.6.

7
- To prevent corrosion and scale formation.
- For effective disinfection.
- Ensure client comfort and minimize risk of skin irritation.

8 Clean the line with the recommended non-foaming cleaner and remove any foam immediately with anti-foaming agents.

9
- Rest or receive further treatments.
- Do not rush nor exhaust yourself.
- Drink plenty of water.

Paraffin wax treatments

1
- Wax treatments are warm and soothing.
- Promote relaxation.
- Relieve aches and pains.
- Soften skin and cuticles.
- Improve stiffness in joints.
- Improve sluggish circulation.

2 When the client has any of the following contraindications:

Skin diseases and disorders	Pustular acne
Cuts and abrasions	Highly vascular
Severe bruising and swelling	Florid, couperose skin

Any nail
infections

Windburn,
sunburn

Any undiagnosed
painful areas

Claustrophobia

3 ■ Burns if the wax is too hot.

■ Cross infection if hygiene standards are not adhered to.

4 49 °C

5 Hands and feet, whole body or face.

6 Tissues are heated:
■ Increase in circulation due to
vasodilation with hyperaemia and
erythema.

■ Sebaceous glands are stimulated
which aids lubrication.
■ The moisture/grease in the wax will
lubricate and soften the skin.
■ Heat soothes sensory nerve
endings.
■ Heat promotes relaxation.
■ Increase in metabolic rate which
improves the condition of the skin.

7 To meet health and safety regulations
all wax must be disposed of after use.
It should be placed in paper, tightly
wrapped and placed in a lined, lidded
bin for collection.

Index

i

Note: page numbers in *italics* refer to diagrams and information contained in tables.